GO
TOWARD
THE
LIGHT

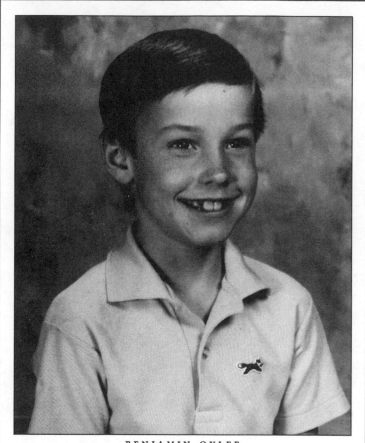

BENJAMIN OYLER

GO TOWARD THE LIGHT

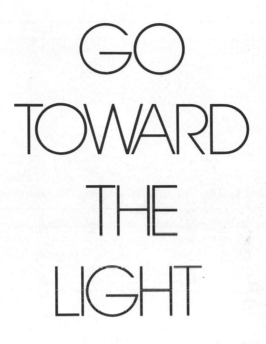

CHRIS OYLER

with Laurie Becklund and Beth Polson

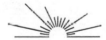

1817

HARPER & ROW, PUBLISHERS · New York

Cambridge, Philadelphia, San Francisco

London, Mexico City, São Paulo, Singapore, Sydney

FIRST EDITION

Designer: *Lydia Link*
Copy Editor: *Bitite Vinklers*

Library of Congress Cataloging-in-Publication Data

Oyler, Chris.
  Go toward the light.

  1. Oyler, Benjamin—Health.   2. AIDS (Disease) in children—Patients—United States—Biography.
3. Hemophilia in children—Patients—United States—Biography.   4. Parent and child.   I. Becklund, Laurie.
II. Polson, Beth.   III. Title.
RJ387.A250956   1988   362.1'96 892'9792 [B] 87-46160
ISBN 0-06-015885-9

---

88 89 90 91 92 CC/HC 10 9 8 7 6 5 4 3 2 1

TO BEN

CONTENTS

1

"Families Are Forever"

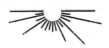

I REMEMBER the numbness that came over me when they told me my seven-year-old son was going to die.

How could this be? He had lived only a short ninety-four months. He had never driven a car. Never gone to a prom. Never held his own child. And now he never would.

Death had always been one of those things that was foreign. And suddenly it was personal. Very personal.

The doctor's words seemed faint behind that deafening hum that filled my ears. The sort of hum that comes from fluorescent lights, only magnified a million times.

It was as if the earth stopped turning on its axis for that moment. I remember thinking how odd it was that the rest of the world kept going on as if nothing had happened. Traffic lights changed color with the same regularity. Birds sat in their favorite trees outside my window and sang their same familiar songs. People laughed and hurried about doing things that didn't really matter.

When you are told that someone you love is going to die, it's as if time skips a beat. And once the clock resumes ticking, nothing is the same. Your voice belongs to a stranger. Your eyes linger on some detail that at any other time would go unnoticed. A smudge on a doctor's glasses. A speck of color amidst other specks of color on a floor.

And in the days and weeks that follow, events that used to approach in some orderly fashion begin swiping at you unexpectedly from the side, keeping you constantly off balance. And when the person who is dying is your child, you know that you will never quite recover. That things will never be the same again. And that the pain will stay inside you forever.

You prepare yourself somehow for the death of someone older. The loss of a parent. Or maybe even the loss of a spouse. But not a child. It seems so much more . . . well, unfair.

At first, we expected a miracle. A change in diagnosis. A cure. Some sort of big, magical eraser from God that would make things right again.

But in the end, it was Ben who let us know that there was no miracle, no magic. That he *was* going to die. And just like the first time he took a step, or rode a bike, or started school, he needed our guidance. Why should this be any different really? Somehow we had to help Ben face death. Without pain. Without fear. And ultimately, without us. Because although we could take his hand and walk with him to the door of death, we also had to stand back then and let him go through—alone. It's the hardest thing any parent could ever have to do—to prepare a child for death and then give him permission to die.

But until that last moment came, I was determined that our family would take every step of Ben's brief but precious journey with him.

But how do you help someone you love die? How could

"Families Are Forever"

I as a mother find the strength to lose my first-born? How could my husband, Grant, deal with not being able to "fix" the biggest problem ever to confront our family? And how could my two other boys, Beau, five, and Aber, three, face losing their hero? All I knew for sure was that we had to do it together.

We took our strength and our hope from the words of a song that we often sang together in our home. Ben knew all the words and always sang them the loudest: "Families Are Forever."

❋ ❋ ❋

That was May 1985. Grant and I had been married for almost ten years. And although we had all the trials and tribulations of any young couple starting a family, we had never encountered sadness, real sadness, before.

We lived in a little duplex in Carmel, California. We had three little boys and it was as if our love grew as our family grew. We never had time to stop and think about being happy; we just were.

Grant worked hard all week. And almost every Sunday, we would come home from church and have a picnic on the lawn. Just Grant and me and the boys. We were so happy, our young family. Sometimes on very sunny, lazy days, the whole lot of us would fall asleep on the blanket after lunch and take a nap.

While other people saved money for a new car or a bigger

house, Grant and I saved money for family trips, little trips to the beach, to the desert, to the mountains. Sometimes we'd camp out and sometimes we'd stay with relatives. Grant and I both grew up in California and both came from large families, six kids in Grant's family, four in mine.

I look back now and marvel at what joyful, carefree times those were. All we wanted was to be together. We were just getting our feet on the ground, just getting our family started, just beginning to enjoy our life. We were so innocent, so naive, so . . . so normal.

＊　　＊　　＊

Grant and I met at church when he was twenty-one and I was nineteen. My mother introduced us.

I remember thinking how good-looking he was and how I wished my eyelashes were as long as his. He was tanned and had a good build, but he was extremely shy. I had been a cheerleader in high school and was more outgoing, so I was the one who ended up doing most of the talking when we first started dating.

We went to baseball games and to the movies and we went for lots of walks around golf courses because golf was Grant's first love. He was truly good, a scratch golfer, and I was convinced that the only reason he was going to college was so he could play on the college golf team.

Grant wanted to be a pro golfer and I was all in favor of

it. I could just imagine myself traveling with him, touring all over the world with my famous husband.

It was on one of our many walks around the golf course in San Clemente, California, where we lived, that Grant and I first started talking about a family. Our family. The family we wanted to have someday.

We wanted eight children. Ideally, four boys and four girls. It was on a long par five that we decided we would name our first son Benjamin.

Then, we laughingly struck a bargain. The deal was that I would raise the children until they were twelve, and then Grant would take over from there so that I could spend some time developing my interest in art.

Funny, but even then I had a terrible fear of someday losing a child. Grant and I talked about it. I told him it was the one thing I knew for sure I could never bear.

Grant gave me a journal as an engagement gift. Inside, he had written the first inscription and had dedicated it to our children. "Today, I gave your mother her engagement ring," he wrote. "Someday I hope you can feel the love that your mother and I have for each other today and the love we will always have for you."

All the journal entries since that day have been mine. I have been the one recording the everyday events of our experience and the joy of our children's births.

Less than two years after we were married, Ben was born. I realized almost immediately that I had never felt quite as close to another human being as I felt to Ben. That there was no bond like the bond between a mother and a child.

But it was also with Ben's birth that I learned that I was a hemophilia carrier. Women carry hemophilia. Men get it. My brother Scott was a hemophiliac and Ben was born with hemophilia too. I soon learned what being a carrier meant. With every pregnancy, the genetic odds would be the same. If we had a boy, there was a 50 percent chance of his being a hemophiliac. And if we had a girl, there was a 50 percent chance that she would be a carrier. So our chances were only one in four of having a hemophiliac child.

But despite the odds, all three of our children, Ben, Beau and Abraham—Aber for short—were born with hemophilia.

When most people think of hemophilia, they think of a cut or an injury where the blood won't clot and the bleeding won't stop. Far more serious and more threatening is an internal bleed—caused by a bruise or an illness. There is a certain protein that is necessary for the blood to clot, and hemophiliacs are missing that protein in their blood. But when they are given highly concentrated doses of the clotting factor they lack, the bleed can usually be stopped. Hemophilia is a disease people can live relatively normal lives with, especially today.

Because of my brother Scott, I had lived with hemophilia, but this was all new to Grant. It was one of the things that made me love him more, just seeing the ease with which he adapted and learned to give the boys their infusions of Factor VIII whenever one them had a bleed.

I loved watching Grant blossom as a father. He was the

kind of father any son would love. And nothing made Grant happier than spending time with his boys. By the time Ben was three, he had already bought him his own set of miniature golf clubs.

Even as a toddler, Ben had a pretty good swing, knocking balls around the backyard. And Grant began to think maybe Ben would be the golfer in the Oyler family.

Grant had given up on his own golf ambitions not long after we were married. I remember exactly how it happened. Grant was talking to some guys on the pro circuit one day, asking them what it was like. They talked about getting a sponsor and a little trailer and pulling it all over the country, from one golf course to the next, hoping upon hope with every tournament, they would finish high enough to earn some cash.

Their description was not exactly the dream Grant and I had in mind for ourselves.

We decided very quickly that that was not the life we wanted for our family, so Grant got a job selling insurance for his father. But that didn't last long. Grant was no salesman.

Not golf, not insurance. But what? Grant didn't know what he wanted to do. Then he heard from a college friend of mine about a contracting job and Grant decided to give it a try.

That's what ultimately led us to Carmel and to Grant's opening his own business. The G. O. Remodel Store, specializing in custom work, remodeling kitchens and bathrooms. I made the sign for the new business and Grant set up shop on the second floor of a hardware store in downtown Carmel.

But getting a new business off the ground wasn't easy. So Grant and I jumped at the chance to go to Park City, Utah, when he had an opportunity to take on a big contracting job there for four months.

It was wintertime. We enrolled Ben and Beau in a wonderful little school there, and they got their first taste of skiing. Aber was still so small that when I bundled him up in winter clothes, he'd walk around like an overstuffed scarecrow.

It was quite an adjustment for all of us when we moved back to Carmel after Christmas of 1984. Grant began working long hours to establish a name for himself and his business. I began helping him out with some accounting and odd projects. Ben and Beau had to leave their friends behind in Park City and start school the second semester in new classrooms in Carmel.

The change was particularly hard on Ben. He had loved his teacher in Park City. She was young and friendly and had brought a feeling of warmth into the classroom. When Ben got back to Carmel, his new teacher was nice enough, but less personal. And he was the only new kid in the classroom. Every day when the school bus arrived, he protested that he didn't want to go to school. I began to worry about him. He just wasn't adjusting well to the change.

So, when we were planning our Easter vacation, Park City seemed like the perfect place to go. The boys could visit their old friends. And our family could spend some time skiing as well.

But I didn't want this just to be a vacation, I wanted it to be a family reunion. I'd been giving it a lot of thought lately. I wanted to bring my own family together for a reunion the way Grant's family did every year.

The Oyler reunions were very special times. There were fourteen cousins by now—Ben was the oldest ("the leader of the pack," everyone called him)—and the reunion was something they looked forward to all year long.

One of the things I had learned in my marriage to Grant was how important the support of an entire family can be, both in good times and bad. Families, when they are close, can provide such a solid foundation for new generations of young families to build upon.

That's what I wanted for my own family, the Eckholdts. But it was much more complicated for us. My parents had gotten a divorce when I was twenty. And, because of our own emotional needs, we had grown apart in different ways. I had remained very close to my mother, less so to my father. I often saw my brother Steve, and even my brother Scott, who was living in Boston. But I missed seeing my big brother Randy, who now lived in Arizona with his wife, Jayne, and two daughters.

My boys didn't even know Randy's girls, Kimmie and Paige. And the girls hadn't been able to spend much time with my mom and Ralph in Los Angeles, either. Ralph Evans was my stepfather. But, more important, he was Grampa Ralph now, one of the greatest grandfathers I could ever have wished for my boys.

Trying to get us all together was a challenge. There were travel plans to coordinate and a few leftover emotional road-blocks to negotiate. And, at the last minute, Scott couldn't make it out from Boston. But finally, we reserved an extra-large condo in Park City and we were ready to pack up.

I was excited, and a little nervous.

Grant took down the boxes of ski gear from the attic and we all dressed up in our ski outfits and began traipsing around as if six feet of snow had just fallen in our living room.

"Look at us, we're hot-doggin'," shouted Beau as he and Ben raced down the hall.

"Remember how much fun we had watching these guys schussboom down the mountain?" Grant asked.

"Even Aber did pretty well at barreling down the hill as long as he could keep his skis straight," I said.

"I liked Aber's stops best," Ben chimed in. "When he was ready to stop, he just fell over sideways." Then, as if on cue, Aber fell over on his back with his skis in midair.

We all laughed. But with the excitement, the laughter quickly turned to giggling. Didn't we look silly, the five of us, ski hats, gloves, parkas, the whole bit, and we hadn't even left the living room.

Getting the boys to bed that night wasn't easy. But finally when they were all tucked in, I asked Grant, "Do you really think it's okay for me to ski? My jumpsuit's already a little tight."

"Just take it easy and stay on familiar runs. You'll be fine."

I was three months pregnant. But we hadn't told anybody yet. We wanted to keep it our own secret, just for a while.

The next morning, we took off before dawn the way we always did on vacation so we could see the sun rise over the highway. The back of the van was loaded with skis and sandwiches and suitcases and little boys asleep in their sleeping bags. I remember thinking as we were driving along that my life was crowded and happy. And I loved it that way.

I've always felt a wonderful sense of well-being in my early months of pregnancy. And that sense was stronger now than ever before, as I realized that my own family was, I hoped, about to be brought back together.

I wish I could say everything fell into place right off. But it had been so long since we were together that everyone was a little awkward at first. We were walking on eggshells that first evening.

The next day I had promised Ben and Beau that we'd take them over to their old school. We had been away four months, but neither Ben nor Beau had been forgotten. Ben's old teacher welcomed him with a hug and the children in his class applauded when he walked in the door.

When we left the school that afternoon, a light snow began to fall and it continued through the night.

The next morning was glorious. The sky was deep, deep blue and the trees were laden with white. I bundled up Aber and dropped him off with the rest of the toddlers in the snow bunny class. Ben and Beau took off in a clatter of skis to line up for class, with Ben showing Beau how to plant his poles so he wouldn't slide straight back downhill.

Steve's a great skier, and he and Grant were a natural pair. So, they took off for the higher slopes while I stayed with Randy. It was hard to believe, but this was the very first time I had been alone with him since I was in high school. He had once meant everything to me. He was the big brother I had looked up to and adored. But we had drifted apart emotionally even before we had stopped living in the same house.

Cautiously, I began exploring how he felt, trying to find out if he remembered the very best times we had ever spent together, when we were small.

"Remember when we were little . . . ," I began as we were riding up on the ski lift. "Remember when you dressed up like a cowboy and your gloves were so long that you couldn't bend your elbows, so I had to walk behind you and draw your gun?"

He laughed. "Yeah, I guess I do."

"You know what, Randy? I loved doing that."

It was my Annie Oakley memories that started to fill in the blank space in our history. It was still hard for us to talk about today, but I knew now we could talk about yesterday. And that was a start.

That afternoon, when we got back from skiing, we all sat around the fire sipping hot chocolate. And then Ben started telling Kimmie about how you could make toboggans out of cardboard boxes. Kimmie hadn't seen a lot of snow, and couldn't wait to go outside and race downhill on Ben's make-shift sleds.

The rest of us stood watching them from the balcony. And just seeing the cousins playing there together, as I had seen the Oyler cousins do at so many family reunions before, made my heart swell.

I stood and watched my boys race down the hill outside the lodge. I was so thankful for them. Their cheeks were all pink from the cold. They had the kind of faces you see on corn flake boxes. Beau with his freckles. Ben with his infectious smile. And Aber with his twinkling, mischievous eyes.

They looked so healthy, so full of life. Beau and Ben were good little athletes. Beau was a soccer player. And Ben could already shoot nine holes of golf. But break dancing was his specialty. We couldn't go anywhere, even to the grocery store, without Ben ending up spinning on the floor—just trying it out.

✳ ✳ ✳

The last day of our vacation started the way many of our days used to when we were children—with my mother making a list.

"I'm making a grocery list for dinner," she said. "Any requests?"

"Chicken wings!" Ben shouted.

"Yeah, chicken wings!" Beau echoed.

Every mother has one special dish that her children love. My mother's was marinated chicken wings. And, even though I used the same recipe, Ben never seemed to like mine as well as Gramma's.

So it seemed especially odd when he didn't touch his food at dinner.

"Hey, Ben, why aren't you eating?" Grant asked.

"My tummy hurts," he answered, looking at me.

"Probably because he ate his chili dog and part of mine too," Beau said.

"Do you feel like you want to throw up?" I asked.

"No, it just aches all over inside."

"Sounds like a touch of the flu," my mom said.

It could have been anything. But I started to wonder what it could be because we were heading back to Carmel and the next day was a school day. Ben had seemed awfully worried about school.

That night when it was time for bed, Aber climbed up on Grampa Ralph's lap for a story. Then Beau climbed up on the sofa beside them. And then Ben. Then Kimmie and little Paige shyly joined the boys. And all their little legs were sticking straight out together, and all their eyes were glistening as Grampa read. I knew then our reunion was a success. There was lots of room to grow. But the trip was an important beginning.

So the ski trip ended. But the stomachache didn't. All the way home to Carmel, Ben wasn't himself. He had started having diarrhea badly enough that I knew I had to call our family pediatrician, Dr. Penn, as soon as we got home.

Dr. Penn would know what to do. He had taken care of Ben since he was born—all the boys, in fact. Dr. Penn didn't look like a doctor, with his cowboy boots and mop of graying hair. And he certainly didn't act like one. He always took time with us—time to take individual interest in the boys and time to include my experience as a mother into the evaluation. But the thing I liked best about Dr. Penn was his calmness.

Because of Dr. Penn's wonderful nature, Ben never had any particular fear of doctors. It was a treat to go see Dr. Penn.

"What's up, Ben?" he asked the morning we arrived in his office.

Once he had heard the symptoms and checked Ben over, it didn't take long for him to come up with a diagnosis. It was probably a parasite, he thought.

"Has Ben been drinking from any private wells?" he asked, trying to find an explanation for his theory. As a matter of fact, he had. We all had. Then why weren't we all sick, I wondered. I guess the rest of us were just lucky. Dr. Penn prescribed an antibiotic for Ben and, just to be on the safe side, took some blood tests too. The results, he said, would be back in a week.

Grant drove Ben to school the next couple of days. Just as Grant stopped the car on the second day, Ben jumped out and ran. He was headed for the bathroom, but didn't make it. He threw up right between two girls. "Ew, gross," one said.

A few days passed and I expected the antibiotics to begin

taking effect. But instead, the diarrhea worsened and the vomiting became more frequent.

On Sunday, Grant had to leave right after church to drive down to Los Angeles to pick up some tiles for his kitchen remodeling business. When he got ready to tell us all good-bye, Ben started to cry. He wanted to go with his dad. Grant wasn't sure it was a good idea, but I pointed out that he wouldn't be able to go to school the next day anyway. And maybe going along would lift his spirits. So the two of them set out for the six-hour drive.

That night, I waited for their call. It seemed like they should have been there already. It had been eight hours. It was late when the phone finally rang.

"Chris, I'm really worried," he said. "Ben's sick, really sick. I don't think this is just a parasite."

I knew Grant. He was doing his best to level with me without scaring me out of my wits.

"What happened? What's wrong?" I asked.

"He had real bad diarrhea and nausea all the way down, and his stomach just hurts him all the time. We got here just a little while ago. We had to stop every twenty minutes."

"Grant, maybe you should take him to an emergency room there."

"He's sleeping now. Why don't you just call Dr. Penn and make an appointment for tomorrow for as soon as we can get back up there, okay?"

"All right, if you're sure."

"He's okay, don't worry. But Chris . . ."

"Yes?"

"I hope you don't mind, but I told Ben about the baby. I thought it might cheer him up. And it did. He was so happy. He promised he wouldn't tell anybody . . . even Beau . . . about his baby brother."

Great. Ben was rooting for another brother.

Early the next morning, we were back in Dr. Penn's office.

Dr. Penn did more tests and said he wanted to call Stanford to talk with them about the symptoms. He said he'd call us at home as soon as he knew anything. We went home but Ben got sicker by the hour. And I didn't know how to help him.

That afternoon, Dr. Penn called to say he thought we ought to take Ben up to Stanford and let them take a look at him.

"We'll leave first thing in the morning," I said.

"Chris . . ."

"Yeah, Dr. Penn?"

"I think you better get ready and go up now."

❋　　❋　　❋

We knew Children's Hospital well because of our annual trips to the hemophilia clinic there. It was a friendly place. Bright. Cheerful. Californian. There were patios and picnic areas. The nurses wore street clothes instead of uniforms.

But being there this time was different.

Ben had lost fourteen pounds in as many days. He weighed less than his five-year-old brother. Every time he ate, he vomited. So, he wouldn't eat. And now in addition to the diarrhea and vomiting, he'd also developed a rash.

I didn't know how much more of this my little boy could stand. I just wanted it to stop. By the time we got up to Stanford, I felt helpless and scared.

The first thing the doctors did was order more blood tests. Lots of blood tests. And one said, "Why don't you go on back home—it'll be a while before we have the results of the tests."

Go back home? That was impossible. I'd watched my son get sicker by the hour for two weeks now. And there was nothing, absolutely nothing I could do to help him. I couldn't . . . I wouldn't . . . take him back home.

"We can't just go home and wait for more test results," I protested. "We've waited a week already. Even Ben's doctor told us to come up here. Right away."

I think the doctors could hear the desperation in my voice because the next thing I knew we were being escorted through double doors to an isolation room. *A private room,* I thought— *wonder how we got so lucky.* Then I realized it had a private bathroom. Of course, Ben needed a bathroom all to himself.

The next two weeks were one big series of tests: stool samples, urine samples, and, of course, more blood samples. I'd never seen so many doctors in my life. And because Stanford is a teaching hospital, every doctor was followed by a gaggle of residents and interns.

At first, I was encouraged by all the activity. Surely, with all this going on, they'd have a diagnosis soon. But each test came back negative and each inconclusive result led to more complicated and more painful tests. A spinal tap. A bone marrow sample. And a brain scan.

Ben was very quiet. I realized I had never seen him afraid like this before. I tried everything to bolster his feelings even though I needed bolstering myself. I read to him, played games with him. I lay on his bed next to him and rub his tummy for hours on end. It seemed to be the only thing that comforted him, and just touching him gave me comfort.

The only time I could get a weak smile out of him was when they came to poke him with another needle and he would start his imitation of Aber, saying, "Be brave. Be brave." That's what Grant and I would say over and over to the boys while we were giving them their factor for the bleeds. But it had become a family joke when we were sitting in church one Sunday and Aber, then just under two, started to pull my hair. When I shrieked in pain, Aber echoed my own advice. "Be bwave. Be bwave."

The slight attempt at humor was the best we could do.

It had already been two weeks and Ben was only getting worse. He had IVs dangling from both wrists. He was in constant pain. And his symptoms seemed to be multiplying. Now he had developed an ugly white coating on his tongue and in his throat and his neck glands were swollen.

There were only two things the doctors knew for sure at that point. One: Ben did in fact have a parasite. And two: his immune system for some reason was not fighting it off.

On Friday, they promised, we would get our first results from the latest tests from the Centers for Disease Control in Atlanta.

The waiting seemed endless. Beau and Aber had gone to stay with Grant's parents, and Grant was commuting four hours a day so he could continue to work and still see Ben and me at night. During the day, it was just Ben and me.

One day, I met another young mother in the hall and we started talking. She had been coming here off and on for five years, she told me. They kept doing tests on her son but they couldn't find out what was wrong with him.

"Five years!" This was beyond my comprehension. "How can you take it?"

"Sometimes not knowing is better than knowing," she answered. "Look around this place. Everywhere you look children are dying. Some have cancer. Some have leukemia. We're lucky."

I thought about what she had said, but I couldn't agree with her. It was the not knowing that was killing me. Not knowing what was wrong. Not knowing what to do. Not knowing when it would end. But what if it were leukemia? The success rate in treating leukemia is high. We could live with that. Anyway, we'd have some answers on Friday.

Grant was working as hard as he could to finish up a job in time to get to Stanford so we could hear the results together. But when Friday came, he called and said he was running late. He'd be there as soon as he could, but he might not make it by the time the doctor came to talk to us.

I watched the clock and I watched the parking lot. No Grant. As much as I hated it I knew I had to go in alone.

"Chris," Dr. Bertil Glader, the head hematologist, said, inviting me into a conference room, "have a seat."

I looked around the room. I was outnumbered. I remember thinking that it didn't take this many people to tell you good news. I could tell by the way they were acting that they had studiously prepared for what they were about to say. And I began to dread hearing their words.

"The results are back, and some are conclusive," Dr. Glader began. "There are other aspects of Ben's condition we're still checking out. Ben does have a parasite. But that's not uncommon in cases like this."

Cases like what? I wondered.

"He also has a swollen gland on the left side of his neck that is responding well to treatment. We're not certain of the cause.

"And he has a pretty serious case of candidiasis. That's the thrush in his throat. But the medication seems to be keeping it under control. Thrush can be very serious if left untreated because it can grow over the throat and effectively stop breathing. But, as I said, it's more or less under control."

Judie Lea, Dr. Glader's nurse practitioner, took advantage of a pause to interrupt. "Chris, would you rather wait for Grant to hear the rest of this?"

"No," I said. *Did they really expect me to leave now and wait some more?* "Please go on."

"Have you ever heard of the acquired immune deficiency syndrome, Chris?" Dr. Glader asked.

Acquired immune deficiency—I repeated the words to myself. *AIDS. He was talking about AIDS.*

"You mean Ben has AIDS?"

"We waited until the results of the tests came back and were conclusive. He tested positive for the HTLV-III virus, Chris. Not just for the antibody. Ben's got AIDS."

Suddenly everything made sense. The private room. The tests sent to Atlanta. The infections Ben couldn't fight off. It was beginning to sink in, even as the doctor went on with his explanation.

Ben could have been exposed to the virus some time ago and it had just been dormant until now, he was saying. Since the factor had been heat treated only for two years, and Ben was seven, he could have been exposed as a baby.

For a fact, Ben had gotten at least two dozen transfusions of the highly concentrated factor a year. And each transfusion contained the blood of at least two thousand donors. That meant Ben had been exposed to the blood of more than forty-eight thousand people a year since he had been born. One of them had AIDS. We had no choice but to depend on all those donors just to keep our son alive. And now, one of them had handed him a death sentence.

I could hear myself asking for details about the disease. Asking about medications. Asking about everything I could think of until Dr. Glader interrupted.

"Chris, do you understand the significance of what we're telling you?"

"Yes," I said. I understood, of course I did—AIDS was fatal. My son was going to die. It was all I could do to form the words to ask, "Can you tell me how long he has?"

"All we know is that statistically eighty-five percent of AIDS patients are dead within a year," Dr. Glader said. "I'm sorry we can't tell you more of what to expect. But Ben's our first."

"He's . . . my first too," I said. "My first son."

I thanked them and accepted their offer to talk to us in more detail once Grant arrived. I wanted to get out of that room. I wanted to get away from the "sentence" they had given my son.

One year—twelve short months. One birthday. One Christmas. One summer. One fall, winter, spring. . . . His words echoed in my ears. "Eighty-five percent are dead within a year."

I needed to touch Ben. To feel the warmth of his breath, to hear his voice call me Mom, to see the weight of his body pressing against the bed. It was an urge much like that I'd felt at his birth—and the birth of all my children—to touch him and examine his body to reassure myself that he was alive and whole. If I hurried, I might reach him before it was official. Before the diagnosis was committed to record that Benjamin Oyler was the first AIDS patient at Children's Hospital.

"Hi, Mom," Ben said when I walked into his room. He was in bed, watching cartoons, totally engrossed, as he was in anything he did. *Of course he was watching cartoons. It was three o'clock. He always watches cartoons at three o'clock. See, things aren't any different. They must be wrong.* I leaned over and kissed him on the forehead and asked if there was anything he wanted. He didn't answer. Just like always when cartoons were on. I took hope from that somehow.

I sat by his bed for a moment. How sunken his eyes looked under those long lashes. Grant's lashes. How narrow his face now, how large his teeth, how wide his mouth. His mouth never used to take up that much of his face. His legs, like skinny little tent poles, were bent and holding up the sheet.

Oh, Ben, why did it have to be you?

I got up and went over to look out the window as my tears began spilling out. How many mothers had stared out at this parking lot before me, crying hidden tears of sorrow over their children? I was one of them now, one of those women the mother with the undiagnosed child would pity.

And then I remembered that conversation Grant and I had on the golf course before we married—that conversation about losing a child. How I knew I could never bear for one of my children to die, that I would go insane, that I would rather die myself. And now it was happening to me. My worst nightmare.

I can't live without you, Ben. I can't. I have spent almost eight years of days full of you. What am I to do if you leave me now? You and I are like an interlocking puzzle. If you take out one piece, the picture falls apart, never to be complete again. I have other boys. I love all of you equally. Yes, equally, but differently. Because each of you is different. And what is different about you, Ben, is that you are most like me. *Whatever is the mortar that binds together a human soul, ours—yours and mine—is the same. The same strength, the same tendency toward private self-doubt. How I've worked on your insecurities, determined that you would overcome them as I never had. I dreamed so much for you.*

I remember when you were just a tiny baby, maybe two weeks old, how I spent one whole day lying on the bed next to you, marveling at your arrival into this world. The sunlight poured through the French doors and your eyes moved around as if there were still just a thin veil between you and this new experience. You were so fresh from God that I wondered if you could still hear angels whispering.

Is it possible that the angels knew even then what you would have to go through? Did they tell you?

I remember how my heart soared when you took your first step. When you said your first word. When you went off to kindergarten that first day with your lunch pail in hand, how I watched you and wondered where the time had gone.

And what about your position as first born? Will it be Beau's first date we remember now? Will it be his going off to college? His getting married?

You can't die, Ben. Not now. You can't die because I can't imagine life without you and if I who gave you life cannot imagine your death, can you die?

I watched Grant's pickup truck pull into the parking lot, past our window and into a parking space. I had to get to him.

I mumbled a weak "Be right back" to Ben. I hurried to

meet Grant but my footing seemed unsure beneath me. The ground seemed to thicken under my feet.

I yearned for Grant's arms around me. Only Grant could comfort me now because only Grant's sorrow could be as great.

I ran the last few yards toward Grant and then buried my head in his chest. I couldn't talk. I couldn't find the words.

"What is it, Chris?"

I started to cry.

"It's AIDS, Grant. It's AIDS."

I could tell by the look on his face that he had known all along. He wasn't surprised. How long had he suspected: A week? Two weeks? How many tiles had he laid and how many long drives had he made alone with his fears, sparing me a few more days of agony?

Tears filled his eyes as he hugged me tighter to his chest. "We'll get through this, Chris. I know we will. I've been praying a lot these last few weeks. I know everything will be all right."

Together we went into a second meeting with the same battery of doctors.

"Any disease, especially chicken pox, could prove fatal," Dr. Glader said.

"Well, at least Ben has had chicken pox," I said. "He's immune to that."

"His immune system is very suppressed," he said. "He is immune to nothing now."

I kept asking about what came next and then next after

that. I needed to know the worst. I needed to know it so I could understand it and so Grant and I could figure out what to do.

They said they would begin by treating the symptoms and then attempt to treat the underlying immune system problem. The rash was already beginning to subside with medication. And the thrush in his throat was somewhat under control with a spray Ben hated but would just have to take anyway. As for the parasite that was causing the worst of his problems, they said they were going to try a new experimental Canadian drug.

Both Grant and I asked a lot of questions about the medication because they told us if we could learn to administer it ourselves Ben wouldn't have to stay in the hospital. That news alone lightened my heart.

We went back to Ben's room immediately after the meeting. I had been gone a long time.

"How are ya, Ben?" Grant asked, giving him a kiss.

"I'm okay."

"It's way past dinnertime, Ben. How about something to eat, something special? Mom or I could go out for anything you want . . ."

"Not now, Dad. Thanks."

Ben didn't know we had seen the doctors, and we didn't tell him. Not yet. Neither of us could face that tonight. Every part of my body felt as though it had been wrung out. I'd slept all week on a cot in Ben's room. But nights were really one long series of trips to the bathroom—not rest. Tonight, Grant was going to stay with Ben. Finally, I said good night and walked over to the Ronald McDonald House alone. It was the first time I had left Ben's side.

The Ronald McDonald House is a lodge of sorts on hospital grounds where family members of patients can rent a room for five dollars a night. In the lobby there is a large, beautiful brass tree, its leaves engraved with names of children who have died. The walls are all painted in cheerful primary colors—and yet it seems lonely. Lonely and sad. Suffering pervades the hallways.

I got into bed in the room they assigned me, but I couldn't sleep.

Images of Ben came spilling into my mind. Ben bringing me bouquets of flowers picked from our neighbor's yard when he was little. Ben giving me a clay heart when he was five years old that said "I love you" across the top. Ben laughing . . . Ben pouting . . . Ben smiling. . . .

I would never, ever erase those images from my memory.

Why Ben? Why Ben? How many times had I asked myself that question? Of all the innocent victims, why did Ben have to get AIDS? It was so unfair! To have hemophilia was a burden enough for a little boy who wanted so much just to be normal, just to play football like the rest of the kids.

Could it be . . . could it be because of something inside Ben that I know, but cannot explain . . . something that has to do with his daydreaming, his determination, his ability to endure. Something I didn't put there. Something that is pure Ben.

Heavenly Father, do You intend to take Ben from me now? Do You need him so? Was it . . . could it have been Your Will that Ben get AIDS? Please bless him, O Lord. He's still just a little boy. He's my son, and I love him. Please don't take him from me.

I turned on the light beside my bed and picked up *Ensign*, a publication of the Church of Jesus Christ of Latter-Day Saints. Grant and I are Mormon, and I usually found something in it to inspire me. But I couldn't concentrate. Too many questions kept racing through my mind, and none of them had answers.

I picked up the phone and called Ben's room.

"Hello," Grant said. His voice was flat.

"You asleep?"

"No, just lying here. Are you all right?"

I couldn't talk so I just held on to the phone and cried.

A few minutes later, Grant came over and got into bed with me. It felt so good to feel his body next to mine, healthy, strong. Lying in each other's arms, we cried.

"Grant," I said after a while, too worn out to cry anymore. "Do you think it's God's will for Ben to die?"

"I don't think it was God's will for Ben to get AIDS, but I know God can make Ben well."

"But what if God's will and our will aren't the same?"

"We don't know that, Chris. Miracles do happen. They do. Maybe all we need is a little miracle. . . . Time. Just enough time for the medicine to work. Just enough time for them to find a cure."

I listened to Grant's words and found strength in them. I

repeated them over and over again to myself. Miracles can happen. They do happen. They *do*.

Faith. Faith and love. That's what we needed now. And we had both in abundance.

The doctors had offered us no hope. So we had to find our own.

2

"*Are There Tacos in Heaven?*"

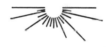

THE DOCTORS HAD DONE all they could for Ben. At least for now. We had come to them with one simple question: "What's wrong with our son?" And they had answered it. But now everything in our lives had a question mark on it. Questions that no one could answer. Questions that would only be answered in time.

For now, we had to learn to live with the questions, to accept them and yet go on.

The doctors had given Ben one year. But what did they know about our family? About our faith? What did they really even know about Ben? Just that he was the first child they had ever had at Stanford with AIDS. As long as Ben stayed in the hospital, as warm and cheerful as it was, he would always remain the little boy behind the double isolation doors. The little boy with AIDS.

I couldn't wait to get him home.

At home, Ben would have his little brothers to cheer him up. The family dog, Darcy, to play with. And both his parents together again, standing by him, no matter what. He could have a bowlful of Chicken & Stars soup and a grilled cheese sandwich for lunch at the kitchen table instead of a ground beef patty and Jell-O on a hospital tray. He could garden with me in the backyard the way he liked to. He could start being Ben again.

I knew it would sound silly to the doctors. But now that I knew what was wrong, I really thought I could help Ben. I didn't think I could cure AIDS. That was up to the medical researchers. But wasn't it just possible that because I was Ben's mother, and knew, as well as anyone knew, how his body worked, that I could help clear up what the doctors referred to as "the symptoms"? The thrush in his throat, the swelling in his neck, the parasite in his stomach. And maybe, just maybe, if I could help fix those problems, then the doctors could concentrate on fixing Ben's immune system.

Maybe Grant was right. Maybe we just needed some small miracles. The patience to hold on without getting discouraged. Time for medical science to find a cure for AIDS. If we could only use all our resources—our family's love, the doctors' dedication, and our faith in God—we could pull Ben through this. Yes, I was beginning to think we could.

Yet I was nervous as we began packing Ben's things to leave. The boxes of toys he had been given. His clothes that were a little too large now. And the medicine, including the precious little pink-and-yellow capsules from Canada that were our most immediate hope.

It wouldn't be easy. I knew that. Once we got home, all there would be was me. Just Chris, twenty-eight years old. That had sounded so old to me on my last birthday. Now it seemed so young, so inexperienced. At least for this. I was a housewife with three little boys and another one—another *baby*—on the way. I never seemed to be able to find enough time now to do the things I needed to. How would I manage when one of my children needed almost constant care? Beau was getting out of school soon for the summer. How would I be able to be a good mother to him and to Aber? How would I be able to take care of myself for the sake of the baby? What in the world would I do when the baby came? How sick would Ben be? What if Ben . . . ?

I tried to rewind the tape in my mind, to erase the what-if questions. I couldn't ask myself those questions now or I would never be able to face the days ahead. I knew I couldn't make the questions go away. But for now, I had to lock them away in my mind where no one, not even I, could get to them.

I knew what my mother would say. One day at a time. Don't get overwhelmed. Just take each day as it comes. That's what I needed to do now.

*   *   *

"Okay, Ben, you can get dressed and go home now," the nurse said cheerfully as she took out the IV that had tethered Ben to a pole for weeks. She spoke so happily, almost as if his illness—like his stay—was over.

"All *right!*" Ben shouted, sliding down off the bed and searching for his tennis shoes. He got dressed and I clipped a brand new pair of suspenders on to his oversized jeans. It hurt him to have anything around his waist.

Ben grabbed his favorite transformer robot from the toy

box and went out ahead of us. He wanted to walk on his own. Grant took my hand and we walked out the double doors and down past the lab, leaving the smell of alcohol and freshly drawn blood behind. Ben called out a quick good-bye to Judie Lea, and we walked out into the sunshine. We were going home.

It was a beautiful early summer afternoon, so we decided to take our favorite route home through the redwoods. It was a two-hour drive back to Carmel, almost twice as long as taking the freeway. But there was no reason to hurry. Beau and Aber were still at Gramma's. Ben lay in the back of the van in the bed we had made him, and for the first few miles, he just looked out at the passing scenery in that dreamlike stare of his—the stare that always made me curious what he was thinking. After a few minutes, he asked to come up and sit on my lap. Before I would have said no, that it was too dangerous. But too dangerous seemed ludicrous now.

He settled in, a little awkwardly around my growing belly, with his head on my shoulder and his feet in Grant's lap.

"What's wrong with me?" he asked. "What did the doctors say?"

Always before I had been able to reassure my boys, saying all those things mothers say to comfort their children. "Everything's going to be fine." Or "It will all work out." Or "Daddy will take care of it when he gets home." But now I didn't know what to say. It wasn't that I didn't want to tell him. I didn't know what to say. There was nothing in my long list of mothering phrases that seemed appropriate.

Grant and I had talked about how we would tell Ben. But we hadn't planned what we would say, the words we would use. We had just made a decision to sit down with him once we were home and be honest with him, the way we always had with our boys. Only this time we had to be careful not to frighten him. And the honest truth by itself seemed too frightening.

"Well, Ben, we should have known Dr. Penn was right about that parasite," I began. "They found one in your stomach. That's why your tummy hurts so much and why you've got all this diarrhea. And the white cakey stuff in your mouth is something they call thrush."

I waited for another question. But Ben was waiting for more of an answer.

"And the reason you're having such a hard time getting rid of all this is because you've got something else too. It's called AIDS. It's a little scary because the doctors don't know much about it yet. You're the very first little boy they've ever seen that has it, Benny."

"When do they say I'm gonna get better?"

"They're not sure, Ben," Grant said. "But the doctors gave us some medicine that's going to make you feel better. Just some pills and some more of that delicious yellow throat spray you love so much. Do you think you can handle that if it'll make you feel better?"

Ben made a face and clutched his throat the way little boys always do when they're pretending to be poisoned monsters from those late-night horror movies.

"If I have to," he said at last. "But I don't understand what I did to get this. Everybody else drank the same water I did. So how come I'm the only one that's sick?"

Grant and I took a moment to plug in that radar parents use to decide who will field a particularly tough question from one of their children. Good. Grant was willing to take this one.

"Well, Ben, it's kind of complicated," he said. "You didn't get AIDS from the water. You got it from the Factor VIII. It's a virus and somebody who donated the blood that they used to make the factor had the virus too.

"Why don't we sit down and talk more about it after you've had a little time to rest up at home? Okay? We're going home now and you're going to be feeling better. So why don't we think up something fun to do, just you and me and Mom?"

"Like what?"

Fun? What did fun mean now? Not skiing or break dancing, not even riding his bike for a while. What sort of fun could we plan for Ben now?

I leaned down and did what I always did when I felt at a loss, when I needed to figure out where to go from here. I pulled out my notebook and a pen from my purse. "Why don't we make a list?" I said.

Grant and the boys were used to my making lists, just like my mom. They probably thought it was in my genes. I made lists sometimes when the demands in my life seemed overwhelming. Writing things down always made me feel organized, even when I wasn't. It helped me divide my life into small, manageable portions. My lists weren't just for groceries but for special things too, because I was always afraid they would get left out. Games to play with the boys. Dream vacations Grant and I wanted to take. Everything on my list was a goal, something to work toward. And when I checked off one of them, I felt good about it, as if I had made a promise to myself and kept it. That's what I wanted to do now, for Ben. To let him dream for a moment, to lay out some goals of his own. Goals that would give him a stake in his own future.

"Let's make a list of things to look forward to," I said. "How about summer? If you had your choice of doing anything you wanted to this summer, anything at all, what would it be?"

"Disneyland!" he said. "Remember, Mom, you said we could go to Disneyland for my birthday when I turned eight. Remember?"

His birthday was in less than a month, June 28. That I remembered. I didn't remember the part about Disneyland. That was Ben's way of laying the groundwork when he really wanted something badly. His strategy was to describe it as if it had already been decided and I had already stamped it with my official mother's seal of approval. It didn't always work. But this wasn't always.

"But even more than Disneyland, I want to go to the Oyler Tahoe family reunion," he said.

Every year Grant's family holds its reunion in Lake Tahoe. But this year it had been canceled because of Ben. Plans were on hold.

"They canceled it because nobody wanted to go without you, Ben," Grant said.

"What a bummer," Ben mumbled.

"Ben, are you up to a reunion?" Grant asked.

"Sure, I love our reunions," Ben said.

"Okay, I'll call Grampa when we get home, and see if we can't work out something."

"That'd be great, Dad! I can't wait to see my cousins."

"What else are you looking forward to, Ben?" I asked.

"Making new friends when school starts in September," he said.

"You might be in a new school, Ben," Grant said. "Mom and I were thinking that we needed to move into a new house before the baby's born in November anyway, and we thought we might try to move before school starts. That way you and Beau can start in a new school with a whole new set of friends."

"Does that mean I can't see Jessica anymore?"

"Of course not, Ben," I said. "You don't have to lose friends just because you go to a different school."

"Yeah, I guess not, not if you really wanna be friends. Can we call her when we get home, Mom, and see if she's feeling better? I'd really like to see her. A lot."

I nodded. But something made me hesitate about putting Jessica's name on the list.

Ben took the pen out of my hand and wrote her name down under new house and new school. J-E-S-S-I-C-A.

"Hey, Ben!" Grant said, changing the subject. "What happens when you turn eight?"

"I get baptized. Write it down, Mom. In capital letters."

B-A-P-T-I-S-M.

"And . . ."

"My birthday party," Ben said. "Lemon cake, Mom. You know, the one with all the lemon stuff drizzled down the side . . ."

Ben looked down at my growing list.

"Something's missing . . . my baby brother."

"You mean Chelsea," I corrected.

Ben gave me a wide smile. He and I knew this dialogue like a familiar storybook. We'd been practicing it at least as far back as before Aber was born. He had wanted a brother then too, and I had wanted a girl.

"Mom, just one more boy, please? I really want another baby brother. I want just one more and then you can have Chelsea. Okay? That a deal?"

We all laughed. Ben was so determined.

"Let's just wait and see what we get. We'll be happy with either one, right?"

Ben looked a little dubious. But he agreed. I wrote "baby" at the bottom of our list and put my notebook away.

I felt as though we had accomplished . . . something. At least we had a plan. A place to start and some signposts that would tell us where we were if we got lost. There weren't any road maps to guide us where we were headed. We would have to find our own way.

*   *   *

Grant began concentrating on the winding road. We were deep into the redwoods now. I could almost reach out and touch the deep red-orange bark of the giant trees as they passed by, one by one. I loved this drive. The forest was so immense, so quiet, it seemed almost sacred. All you could see was giant trunks reaching way up to the sky with just a little patch of blue over the treetops.

We drove along quietly, just feeling content for the moment to be together in this beautiful forest. I had to learn to appreciate these moments now, each of them, and not look forward and not look back. Because nothing was going to be the same, at least not for a while. And I didn't know if the future was our friend or our enemy.

*   *   *

That night Ben slid deep down into the familiar smell of his own sheets and slept. Soundly, as when he was a baby and fell asleep with his worn yellow blanket. He slept most of the next two days, too. On the third morning, I was making breakfast when I heard the patio door slide open, and Ben's voice asking if he could go outside and play with our basset hound, Darcy. "Sure, honey, but breakfast is almost ready," I answered.

"Are There Tacos in Heaven?"

It took me a moment to realize how *normal* that conversation was. Before I had taken it for granted. Now, normalcy felt so good, so comforting. Normalcy meant nothing less than life itself. I couldn't wait to pick up Beau and Aber. By evening, our family would finally be together again.

Beau and Aber had been at my mother's in Los Angeles. Mom and Ralph were going to drive them up to San Luis Obispo and we'd meet them there. Ben had been resting for two days, and I thought he looked a lot better. I was encouraged until I saw the shock on my mother's face. She and Ralph hadn't seen Ben since those first tummyaches in Park City. That had been less than two months before. But it seemed like another lifetime now. When we drove off, I saw Ralph put his arm around my mother's shoulder.

Going home, the backseat of our van was filled with little boys' laughter. Our boys. Three of them. Thrilled to be together. Ben was already into the treats Beau and Aber had brought back from Gramma's house. For now, their laughter was enough.

The next day, while Ben was taking a nap, Grant and I talked to Beau and Aber and told them that Ben was still sick, very sick, and that he needed to rest a lot more than he used to. But we didn't go into the details of AIDS. There seemed little point.

Grant had to get back to work. He had missed so much time while he was up at the hospital that he was going to have to work fourteen-hour days just to meet the deadlines for the remodeling contracts he had signed. But when he left the house, I felt suddenly alone. Always before, when there was a big challenge in my life, I would talk it out with someone. Grant. Or my mother. Now there was no one to talk to because no one knew any more than I did.

Those early weeks were a difficult time for all of us. I told myself that we were going through the hardest part, getting used to this new way of living, even getting used to looking at Ben—the new Ben. Still so thin and pale. I told myself that it would get easier. That every day the improvement in Ben would be so slight that it would be almost impossible to detect. I told myself not to make too much of the good signs, Ben keeping down a whole sandwich at lunch, Ben riding his bike down the block, because if I acknowledged those, I would have to acknowledge the bad signs as well. Ben's diarrhea. Ben's vomiting. Ben's fatigue.

It was a daily battle. The alarm would ring at 6:00 A.M. and Grant would get up and go into the bathroom to take a shower, and I would just lie there. I was four, almost five, months pregnant. I needed my rest. That's what I told myself. But what I really wanted was just to pull the covers over my head and make the past few weeks go away. I just couldn't shake off the feeling that it was all a mistake. That this wasn't supposed to be happening. Not to Ben. Not to us. That somebody had put the wrong zip code on this package and delivered it to the wrong address.

What had we done to deserve this? Why had this dark cloud come to park right over our little house when I could look out and see sunshine right there, right across the street?

I wanted to cry. I wanted a time machine to take me out of here, to take me back where things were the way they used to be.

Then Grant would come out of the shower and kiss me, and sometimes put his hand on my stomach to see if he could feel the baby kicking, and remind me just to take one hour, one day, at a time. He would tell me he loved me and that together we would pull through this. And I would think, *Yes, it will be all right. As long as Grant believes it, it will be.* He was my rock in this storm, my promise that somehow, no matter what happened, he would help me through it.

So, I would get up, thinking maybe it was lucky I had to get up because facing the day ahead was easier than staying in bed and facing my fears. And the day ahead was hard enough.

School was out now, and Beau was home with his own social and athletic schedule. Aber was his usual rambunctious little self, a three-year-old intent on getting into everything. And Ben required almost constant attention. His diarrhea never stopped. We were living in a two-bedroom, one-bathroom duplex, and Ben had to be in the bathroom every hour or so all day long and sometimes all night as well. He began carrying a little U-shaped basin around with him because he was still vomiting frequently, and sometimes he couldn't quite make it to the bathroom. So suddenly I had five loads of laundry a day.

I had hoped somehow to make up for all this sickness and hard times with special trips and outings for the boys. I had pictured myself having tender heart-to-heart moments with

Beau and Aber and, of course, Ben. But I couldn't figure out a way to do it between twenty-four-minute wash cycles and medicine dosages and spur-of-the-moment trips to the grocery store when there was something Ben actually felt like eating and we didn't have it.

My big challenge got consumed by a series of minor, irritating little challenges. Hygiene, for example. We weren't afraid anyone would catch AIDS from Ben because we had learned it is transmitted almost solely through sexual intercourse or other exchanges of body fluids, such as blood transfusions. But the other problems, especially the thrush in Ben's throat, were contagious. I had to be particularly careful around Ben because I was pregnant and handling fluids from his body. We put liquid soap dispensers and paper cups in the bathroom. But it was hard enough just keeping track of Beau and Aber, let alone making sure they weren't eating off Ben's Astropops popsicle.

One of the hardest parts was the fact that the boys weren't always getting along as well as they had before. It started with the toys Ben had been given at the hospital. Wonderful battery-operated cars and robots with lights for eyes, the kind of toys every child always wants for Christmas. Beau and Aber were getting into little fights over them. Sometimes Ben would play peacemaker. But other times he would just be so tired that he'd put his hands over his ears and order them out of his room. That only caused more problems, because it was their room too, and their feelings got hurt. We needed a bigger house. Soon.

I tried hard to take the boys out, to plan a trip to the aquarium or the park. But some days Ben wouldn't be up to it or sometimes he would feel all the worse for being in a place where other kids were laughing and having fun. So, more and more, Ben and I did one-on-one things together. We would garden or make paper masks. Or, sometimes, when Ben was feeling tired and I was exhausted with worry and with the pregnancy, we would just lie down together on the living room floor and take a nap. I had not had times like that with Ben since he was little. It was those quiet moments, sweet moments with Ben, as rare as they were, that enabled me to get through those early weeks.

Things that had been a part of my regular activities now seemed like a welcome relief. Working with the class of teenaged girls at church. Keeping the books for Grant's business. Making a stained glass window. Anything that for one brief hour could take me out of my role as a mother of a dying child.

Before, our family had gone out to dinner maybe once a week. We had stopped because Ben had such a hard time eating. But he still enjoyed the outings, so one night Grant asked him to choose his favorite restaurant. He chose Plaza Linda, and we went. He ate a whole taco and part of a burrito. But when he started coughing, the kind of thick, deep cough that comes only from someone very, very sick, the other customers turned and looked. There was this little boy with a basin in his lap.

They were wondering—I know they were—what was

wrong with Ben. I just wanted to stand up and tell all those people that there was nothing at all wrong with Ben. That he hadn't done anything wrong. That it wasn't his fault. That he was only seven. And that he used to be just Ben and he still was, inside. But I didn't say anything. Neither did Grant. Instead, we just felt uncomfortable and embarrassed. We ate quickly and left. Going out to eat was the first item on a new list. Of things not to do.

But one morning, as I was squirting Ben's throat with the yellow medicine he hated, I noticed that the swelling in the gland in his neck was gone. I was ecstatic.

"Ben!" I cried out. "Your neck is better!"

"I know, Mom. It's been better for a couple days," he said nonchalantly. "Does that mean you don't have to spray that awful stuff down my throat anymore?"

"Afraid not, honey. That's for the white stuff in your mouth. You know, it looks like that's getting a little better too."

Ben was scheduled for a checkup the next day at Stanford. I had been dreading it. But now I couldn't wait to hear the good news.

They gave Ben a gamma globulin shot as soon as we got up there, and Grant and I were encouraged. Gamma globulin was for his immune system. They were beginning to work on his immune system. The doctor's report noted that the swelling in Ben's neck was gone. There was progress.

As we left the hospital, Aber asked, "Mommy, is Ben all better now?" I don't remember what I answered, but it was the first of many times to come that Aber would ask me that question.

I was at the grocery store later that day when I bumped into Ben's school bus driver, who told me Jessica had died a few days before. The first thought that crossed my mind was that I had let Ben down. I hadn't called Mrs. West since we'd gotten home. And now it was too late. What would Ben say? How would he handle this, now?

Jessica was really a very special friend to Ben. He had gotten to know her one day when he had to stay inside from recess in the first grade because he had a bleed. Jessica, "the girl with no hair," was there too. She had explained to him that her head hadn't always been like that, that it was just since they had found tumors in her brain and had started chemotherapy that her hair had fallen out.

Ben understood that Jessica would probably die someday. Grant and I had talked to him about it one night after Jessica's mother had called. She, too, had seen how close they had grown, and she didn't want Ben to be hurt. That was almost two years ago. Now, everything was all topsy-turvy. How would I tell Ben?

I decided to take the boys to the park the next day. The park with the giant slide that Ben loved so much. He couldn't climb the steps now, but he still enjoyed the swings and some other things.

We sat down on the edge of the sandbox. Beau and Aber played nearby.

"I have to talk to you about Jessica, Ben," I said.

He looked up at me quickly, and then looked down and started doodling in the sand with his finger.

"It's not good news, is it?"

I put my arm around his shoulder. "No, it isn't, Ben. Jessica died a few days ago."

He kept tracing something, a circle, in the sand.

"You know, Mom, I really loved Jessica. She was my best friend. There was nobody else I ever knew that understood me like Jessica at school. Not even the boys. I'm really gonna miss her. . . .

"Why did I have to lose her so fast, Mom? She wasn't even as old as me."

I didn't know what to say. I didn't know the answer. I didn't seem to know the answers to a lot of things anymore.

"You never have to lose somebody you really love, Ben," I began. "You can keep them with you, always. In your heart."

I took out my wallet and showed him the pictures I kept in there of him and Beau and Aber and Dad. "Did you know your heart can take pictures? And they're the best kind because you take them at the most special moments. And nobody has those same pictures but you."

"Will Jessica go to heaven?"

"Yes."

"Will I see her again someday?"

"I'm sure you will, Ben."

There was a long silence. Ben just kept looking down and drawing in the sand.

"When will that be, Mom?"

"I don't know, Ben. Nobody knows exactly when they're going to die. That's why it's so important to love each other while we are together."

I kept my eyes wide open so the tears wouldn't spill out. Why did I have the feeling that he knew he was dying? That despite our careful words and assurances, he had understood it all. Why did I have the feeling that he wanted to talk to me, too. But he couldn't because he was afraid of scaring me.

I just wanted to hold him tight and rock him back and forth in my arms and cry with him. For our suffering. For his pain. For the years we might not have together. But I couldn't because I was afraid of scaring him.

So we sat there. Ben with his thoughts. And me with mine.

"Mom," he asked finally. "Will you push me on the swings for a while?"

"Sure, Ben."

Playing with Jessica was one thing on Ben's list he would never do. But he did go to Disneyland that summer. He was very excited. We all were. Grant's father had pulled together a reunion in record time, arranging for six families to meet at Disneyland.

I had always admired Grant's father for his strength. I thought of him as a kind of patriarch, strong-willed with white hair, the kind of man who always did what he set his mind to. He and Grant's mother had had six children. Grant was their fourth child, but their eldest son. And Grant's son Ben was the first of their fourteen grandchildren. I knew that Grant's parents held a special love for Ben.

But, for reasons we didn't understand, Ben was much weaker by the time we went to Disneyland.

He went on as many wild rides as he could. And then, he and Grant went off alone to spend all the rest of their tickets at the Frontierland Shooting Arcade. Ben was too weak to hold up the heavy rifle, so Grant held it for him, and Ben pulled the trigger.

The next afternoon, we all gathered around the motel pool. All the cousins were splashing in the water, and Ben was just sitting in a deck chair, watching. None of his cousins was talking to him. It wasn't their fault. They were just little. And Ben probably didn't look like Ben to them anymore.

I sat with Ben until Beau came over and asked me to take him to the Jacuzzi. Children weren't permitted in the Jacuzzi alone.

As Beau lowered himself into the warm bubbles, I looked back to keep an eye on Ben. There was a glass divider with a metal rim between me and him. It was like looking at him in a picture frame. And suddenly, from this spot, I saw Ben the way everybody else saw him. A pale, emaciated, sickly little boy with hollow cheeks. A little boy wrapped in a blanket and still shivering even on this hot summer day.

I couldn't believe that boy was Ben. My Ben. Right at his feet, the pool was crowded with healthy, normal kids who were probably playing a game Ben had taught them the year before. What had happened to the "leader of the pack"? Why wasn't he out there organizing underwater swim races or running across the slippery deck despite my warnings, or doing cannonballs into the pool?

Why did it have to be Ben? Why? It wasn't that I wanted any other child to get it. But why Ben? That question would never leave me. Every time I looked up to see Ben, this new reality struck me. Clearly, without a doubt, Ben did have AIDS. And Ben was dying. And no matter how hard I tried, no matter how much I wanted it, the old Ben wouldn't come into focus in that frame. I sat and I cried. I can't even remember how long. Nobody could see me back there. Even Beau had gone back to the pool.

Finally, Grant came looking for me. He sat down beside me and looked out the glass at Ben, and then over at the kids in the pool, and tears came into his eyes too.

I could see anger and sorrow and frustration written on his face. He was crying because it hurt him so much to see Ben suffer. I was crying because I knew in my heart that the doctors were right, that Ben did have AIDS and that he *was* dying. I accepted those things as facts. I knew now that it really would take nothing less than a miracle to save Ben. But what if there wasn't a miracle for Ben? There it was again. What if . . . ? I tried to close the door to those what-if questions that were clamoring to get out. Did Grant have those what-if questions inside too? As hard as I looked, I couldn't see them written on his face. And I couldn't bring it up. I couldn't ask him. Not any more than he could have told me when he first suspected Ben had AIDS.

It was a new feeling for me, not sharing my innermost

thoughts with Grant. The biggest secret I had ever kept from him before was what I had gotten him for Christmas. This disease was affecting us in ways I had never guessed. It was showing Grant and me to be very different people. I, the practical one, who needed to know the worst to go on. Grant, the believer, who had enough faith to carry on in the certain belief that Ben would live. Each of us would have to cope with this trial in our own way and draw strength from each other. Like when Randy and I were little and we used to roller-skate down the sidewalk with a rope between us, and he would hurl me fast ahead of him so I could turn around and whip him up ahead of me again. That way we kept propelling each other ahead, inventing energy, where there was none before. That's what Grant and I had to do for each other now.

Soon after the reunion, we took Ben back to the hospital. In the van on the way, Ben asked me about his baptism. His birthday was in another week, and he could be baptized as soon as he was eight. "As soon as you're feeling better," I told him, "we'll set up the baptism."

Once he was hooked up to the IV again, Ben began gaining weight. He had grown dehydrated from all the diarrhea, that was all. After only a week, we went back home with Ben looking more like Ben again. This time we took the freeway. It was faster. And it was Ben's birthday.

We had a quiet picnic on the lawn, the way we used to on Sunday afternoons. My mom and Ralph were there. Ben ate every bite of his lemon cake with "all the lemon stuff drizzled down the sides." And he blew out all the candles on the first try. I wondered what he wished for. But I didn't ask and he didn't tell me.

"Is Ben all better now, Mommy?" Aber asked.

"Hey, watch this, Aber," Ben said.

Ben got up and poised himself on the slick floor of our entryway just inside the door. Ben the break-dancer. He was aiming for a backspin. Usually he'd go around four or five times at a try. This time he stopped himself after two and just lay there, crushed.

"It hurts, Mom," he said.

"What hurts?"

"My bones. My bones just hurt."

I told him he was still the best little break-dancer in my book and helped him up. I was about to take him inside to rest, when he called out to Aber.

"You been practicing like I taught you, Aber?"

Aber toddled up and got down on the floor, proud as could be to perform for Ben. He wobbled through a kind of spin on his back, his little canvas high-tops kicking wildly in the air.

"That's great, Aber," Ben said with a private smile for me. "Next time, hold your arms tighter."

That night when we tucked Ben in, he said, "I'm eight now. Remember what happens when you turn eight?"

I had been putting it off. Ben's baptism. I just had this feeling, this fear, that once Ben was baptized he would somehow be ready to die. That he would be one step closer to God and one step farther away from me. It was silly. I knew that. What did I think I was doing? Fighting some sort of tug-of-war with God for the life of my son? God was on my side.

Ben's illness had started to reach deep into parts of my life that I didn't want touched, that I had sacrificed to build. My relationships with my children. My marriage. My faith.

Grant made arrangements with the church for the baptism. But because Ben had AIDS, we had to get special permission to use the font at the church. Finally, the word came from the president who resided over our ward and six other church wards. The janitor would have to bleach the font before and after Ben was baptized. But we could use it. Another thing on Ben's list was going to happen.

The next night we sat down for what we as Mormons call a family home evening. It's an important tradition to us. It's a time when we turn off the television and disconnect the telephone. It's a time when we focus on our family and our faith.

We tell stories. And we sing songs. It's like a family council where any member of the family, either a child or adult, can bring up something that is bothering him as an individual or something we need to discuss as a family. Little gripes and big growing pains get handled here.

This particular night we would talk about Ben's baptism. We all gathered in the living room around the fire. Grant sat on the couch with Aber next to him. Ben and Beau and I sat on the floor.

"It's a pretty big day in your life," Grant began. "Do you know what happens?"

"You get dunked!" Beau said. Ben looked at him with just the slightest bit of impatience.

"That's right," Grant said. "But do you know what it means?"

"It means you're making promises to our Heavenly Father and He's making promises to you," Ben said. Ben had studied about baptism in Sunday school.

"It's kinda like joining God's football team," Grant said. "And it means you want to play real hard for Him. And He's going to help you be a really good member of the team because He's going to give you a coach . . . do you know who that coach is?"

"The Holy Ghost," Ben said.

Aber perked up. "A real live ghost?"

"You can't see the Holy Ghost, Aber," Grant answered. "But He's always there. And you can hear Him talk to you if you listen really hard. It's not like our voices. It's just a quiet little voice inside your head. And if you listen carefully, He will always tell you right from wrong.

"And you can tell when you've done something that's really right because it'll feel all warm and fuzzy inside, like someone is tickling your insides and making you feel good.

"There is something else the Holy Ghost does too. And it's very important. He's a great comforter. If you're not feeling well or are feeling a little down, the Holy Ghost will comfort you. That will be important to you, Ben, when you're feeling real sick. You could use some comforting, couldn't you?"

"Yeah, Dad. But, you know, I was wondering about something."

"Yes?"

"Are there tacos in heaven?"

Tacos in heaven. We all laughed out loud.

"That's a tough one, Ben. You know there are lots of things we don't know exactly. We just have faith that things in heaven will be warm and comforting."

"Do people live in houses in heaven?"

"They all live in God's house, Ben," Grant said. "We don't know exactly what it looks like. But it will feel like coming home. You know what it feels like to get back home after you've been away for a while? You know how good it feels. That's what it will feel like . . . like going home."

Ben asked more questions. Are there trees in heaven? What about streets? How long does it take you to get there? How do you get around once you're there? They were questions that touched me for their innocence, and then disturbed me because they were so practical.

The next morning, Ben drew a poster in orange and pink felt pen. On one side, he wrote the three promises God would make to him, and on the other, the promises he would make back. "I promise," he wrote in fancy letters, "I will remember Jesus. I will keep his commandments. I will help others." On the other side, he wrote: "My Heavenly Father *promises:* He will forgive us. He will give us the help of the Holy Ghost. He will help us to be happy."

I watched Ben from the doorway of his room as he tacked the poster on the wall.

"Being baptized is a big responsibility," I said. "You know that, Ben?"

"Yes."

"It means that from now on you're going to be responsible for your own actions."

Ben just looked at me as if he already knew everything I was saying.

"Are you ready for that responsibility?"

"I am, Mom. I know I am."

Ben was ready to be baptized. I had to get ready too.

When the day arrived, my father and his wife, Marilyn, came for the ceremony. That meant so much to Ben. And to me. We didn't see them often enough, but there's something about having your family together at special times that makes everything feel so complete.

Ben listened, really listened, to every word of the ceremony. He never once took his eyes off the bishop. He seemed so grown up.

AIDS had made me aware that the human body is capable of unbelievable physical change. I had seen it, in Ben, in the past few weeks alone. Now I was becoming aware that the soul, too, could change. Even in a little boy.

After it was over, I walked up to Ben with a towel. He was just standing there, dripping wet in white pants and a white shirt. He hugged me and said, "I love you, Mom." He was so skinny, I felt as though I could see his soul shining through his body. And it filled the room.

I will never forget how he looked standing there, like a powerful but very skinny little angel. His body was shrinking. But his soul was growing. My heart took a picture.

3

"Will You Be Mad at Me
if I Die?"

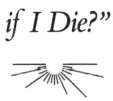

I WASN'T SURE when it happened, but somehow time began passing again. June turned into July. And the fog rolled in the way it did every summer in Carmel.

We found a bigger house—one with two bathrooms. Grant closed the books on one of his remodeling jobs and was trying to catch up on others. Beau lost two baby teeth. Aber outgrew his Hot Wheels and got a bike with training wheels. I finished a stained glass project and packed away my tools, not knowing when there would be time to use them again.

And Ben, Ben had good days and bad days. On the good days, we cherished every laugh and every smile. On the bad days, we longed for the good days.

In a way, creating a life for Ben was a lot like working on my stained glass projects. We took every little odd piece of time and every bright moment we could find and tried to make something beautiful.

There was no way to compensate for Ben's suffering. No way to put a normal eight-year-old's life into Ben's frail, weak little body. But we tried.

There was unlimited frozen strawberry yogurt, Ben's new favorite. And an unending number of trips to Oscar Hossen-fellder's, an amusement park on Cannery Row in Monterey. It was like Las Vegas for children. Loud music and cheap prizes. Cotton candy and salt-water taffy. Arcade games and a magic shop. And Ben loved it all.

He was still good at the arcade games, especially Skee Ball, but he wasn't as interested in the prizes as he used to be. He gave his winning tickets to his brothers so they could pick out the plastic trick of their choice.

There were moments that just a few months ago had seemed ordinary. Now they seemed special.

We tried not to dwell on the word *AIDS*. To keep it a term we used just with doctors, at the hospital. But it found its way into our home anyway. Through the television, the newspaper, and conversations with friends.

Beau was just a kindergartner when Ben got sick. He was just beginning to learn to read. But he knew the word *AIDS*. I found that out the afternoon he lost a front baby tooth. I had been so busy with Ben, I hadn't even realized his tooth was loose.

He came running in to me with his tooth in hand, informing me that he was going to put it under his pillow, even though he knew I was really the tooth fairy. I pretended to have no personal knowledge of the tooth fairy's activities, and wrapped up some ice in a cloth diaper to control bleeding. Grant would be home for dinner soon and we could give Beau his shot of Factor VIII.

I had given the boys shots. I did it often. But I was still a little squeamish about sticking the needles in my children. And Grant always seemed to have such a sure hand.

When Grant had asked me to marry him, I remember

telling him with some apprehension that there was a possibility that I might be a carrier. "It doesn't matter, Chris," he told me. And it really didn't.

When Ben was born a hemophiliac, we were so joyful just to have him that we felt as though we were consoling Dr. Penn when he told us the results of the hemophilia test. "It'll be all right," I said. "Just don't circumcise him."

I remember writing in my journal that if wars came, as they seemed to every generation, I would never have to send my son off to fight.

Ben's first major bleed happened when he was just eight months old and he cut his lip trying to stand up by the dishwasher. We took him to the hospital, and he screamed his little lungs out while Grant and I held him to keep his arms down so Dr. Penn could give him the first shot. It seemed so cruel. It hurt so much just to watch the needle go into his scalp, because that's the only visible vein they could find. And that was just the beginning.

By the time Ben was four, there had been a lot of advances in the treatment of hemophilia. The most important was home treatment kits. It meant that we could take care of the bleeds at home instead of running off to the hospital every time there was a cut or a bump or a fall. It saved time and money. But most of all, it made us feel self-reliant, that we could take care of our own children.

Home treatment was possible because medical science had developed a way to extract the factor that hemophiliacs were missing from whole blood. So, instead of getting transfusions of whole blood from one donor, which wasn't always enough to stop the bleed, they were given concentrates of the factor from blood of many donors, thousands of donors.

It was those advances that had made hemophilia manageable. That was the word I used. Manageable. It meant keeping a supply of Factor VIII on hand, in the refrigerator. And it meant dropping everything when the factor was needed.

There was an attitude about hemophilia that had become second nature to us. We knew to buy the boys baseball mitts instead of football helmets, bicycles instead of roller skates. We wanted to be protective enough but not overly protective. We never wanted our boys to grow up with fears, with emotional scars as a result of their physical limitations.

I remember the day Ben's kindergarten teacher sent home a picture of Ben on the playground slide. He had his eyes wide open and his arms outstretched as he took the plunge. She pinned a note to the picture saying that Ben was the least fearful, most adventuresome kid in the whole class. I was so proud of that. So proud of how the boys were learning to take their disease in stride.

But, for some reason, Beau was nervous that night as Grant was drawing the factor up into the syringe.

"You're letting some bubbles in, Dad!" he said. "Don't let any bubbles in!"

"Don't worry, Beau, you know the bubbles won't go inside," Grant said.

"Please, Dad. Be careful, please!"

Grant put down the syringe and asked Beau what was

wrong. Beau just looked real scared, and tears were welling up in his eyes.

"I don't wanna get AIDS. I don't wanna get AIDS like Ben did from the bubbles," he said.

We couldn't figure out just why Beau thought AIDS lived in the bubbles. While Grant explained to him that there was no AIDS in the bubbles, I picked up the Factor VIII and showed him the letters *H.T.* on the box.

"See, Beau, look at the letters," I said. "*H.T.* That stands for heat-treated. That means that the factor in this bottle has been heated until it was very, very hot to kill any AIDS germs that might have been in there. And we use only factor that has been heat-treated . . . so you don't have to worry."

Until that moment, it hadn't even occurred to me that Beau might have been exposed to the AIDS virus too. Why hadn't it? I guess I had been so worried about Ben that I didn't have room for any more worries.

Beau had been born in 1979, four years before they started heat-treating the factor. The fact was he could have been exposed to AIDS. But realistically, the odds were overwhelmingly against it. Besides he wasn't sick.

And Aber was probably safe. They had started heat-treating factor soon after he was born. But I decided to have both of them tested—for my own piece of mind.

*   *   *

I was only three years old when my brother Scott was born with hemophilia. Every time he had a bleed, he would have to go to the hospital for a week of transfusions. My brother Randy and I would sit downstairs in the lobby of the UCLA Medical Center with coloring books and crayons because we were too young to go upstairs to Scott's room.

I have such vivid memories of sitting in that lobby, hour after hour, day after day, waiting for my mom and dad.

In addition to the hemophilia, Scott had also been born with glaucoma and he had had to have a number of operations on his eyes. When he was two, they couldn't stop the bleeding in his eye after an operation and he lost the sight in one eye.

When Scott started to lose the sight in his good eye, the doctors had to operate again.

I remember when he came home from the hospital that time. He was sitting on the floor in the living room with bandages over his eyes and he was crying. He wanted to take the bandages off so he could see how to play. But he couldn't.

Randy and I were sitting on the couch.

"How come I can't be like the other kids, like Chris and Randy?" Scott asked. "When will I be able to play again?"

And then my mother sat down and took Scott's hand. I will never forget the sound of her voice, how quietly and how calmly she talked to him. And I'll never forget what she told him.

"You know, Scott, there are all different ways to see. We use our eyes because it's the most convenient. But we can also see with our other senses. We can learn to see with our touch, our taste, our hearing, our smell."

Scott listened. So did Randy and I.

"Scott, when we take the bandages off this time, it's going to be different. This time you're not going to be able to see with your eyes.

"But you're going to learn to see in other ways. And I'm going to help you."

She held Scott in her arms and she cried. Randy and I cried too. Scott's life would never be the same again.

I never forgot that moment. The courage that my mother had. The strength she gave Scott.

Somehow she made it sound like an adventure. That Scott was going to learn to see in all sorts of magical ways that other little boys and little girls couldn't do. With his hands. With his ears. With his heart. And most of all, he would have her there to help him, every step of the way.

After Ben got sick, I began to see that memory differently. Not as a little girl, but as a mother. Where did my mother find the right words to say to Scott when, as I realize now, she must have been suffering so much herself? Where did she find it in her imagination to tell Scott the way around an obstacle at the same time she told him about the obstacle itself? And how did she know to help Scott find the beauty ahead of him, even in the darkness?

Whatever she had given him, it had worked. In spite of his blindness and his hemophilia, Scott had gone to college, gotten a job, and was living on his own. He was fiercely independent but always the first one to offer his help. When Ben had been diagnosed with AIDS, Scott was one of the first to call.

He had come such a long way since my mother told him he was going to be blind. He was only eight then. Eight. Ben's age.

Would I ever be able to do that for my own son? Would I ever be able to reach down inside myself and find some magical words that would make everything feel right, even when we knew everything was so wrong? Where was I supposed to begin looking? Did I have it inside me to find?

What could I give Ben, what inspiration, what prize, what goal, that would be worthy for him to work toward? What would make him want to keep living through pain and what the doctors had said was certain death?

How could I possibly help him look forward to the future when what I really wanted myself was to take the hands of the clock and turn them backward? Backward to whatever that day was when Ben had gotten his fateful injection, to a moment when I could undo what had been done.

But I couldn't. There was no way.

And that was where the anger stepped in and replaced the fear.

Anger was a pretty foreign emotion to me. Sure, I got mad at little things every now and then. But that emotion came and went. That wasn't anger. That was getting mad.

Anger was something I observed in other people. People

who threw things and swore at other people in their cars. I didn't do those things. Not me. But I began to realize that one of the emotions that was rising up inside me was, in fact, anger. And I didn't want to feel it at all because it didn't serve any purpose, and because I didn't like the way it felt, like wearing somebody else's clothes.

I didn't know it at the time, but I was just the first in our family who was going to have to learn to deal with anger. Everyone else would too, sooner or later. Ben had so clearly been wronged. I wanted someone or something to blame. But what good would it do?

I wasn't angry all of the time. I really wasn't. It was just that it kept cropping up from time to time when I least expected it, at times when I wasn't thinking about AIDS at all, and something would happen to remind me it was still there.

Like the night Ben came into the kitchen with a question while Grant and I were making dinner.

"Dad, what does *gay* mean?" he asked.

Oh, Ben, I thought. Please don't ask this. It's so unfair to make you have to go through this too, on top of everything else. Do we really have to put this on your shoulders as well?

"Why do you ask that, Ben?"

"Because I heard it on TV. They said on TV that God is going to punish all the gays with AIDS."

"They're not talking about you, Ben," I said. Grant and I looked at each other.

"Why don't we all go in the living room?" Grant said. Beau and Aber were outside playing. Dinner could wait. But

Ben's question couldn't. We needed to talk about this now.

Last year, Grant had sat down with Ben in just the same way to talk to him about sex after he had come home from school with some dirty word he didn't understand. We hadn't planned to talk to him about sex yet, but we didn't want him to think it was a dirty joke either. So, Grant had explained just enough for him to understand how babies were made, to understand that sex was a normal part of a husband and wife loving each other.

That talk had made sense. Then.

And now Ben had good reason to ask about homosexuality. He was suffering from a disease the television said was a gay disease, tied to the homosexual community. So he wanted to know what *homosexual* meant, what *gay* meant.

Pretty soon he would be back in school, and he would undoubtedly hear more. I guess we had to explain. At least enough so he didn't feel we were keeping a secret from him. At the same time, it seemed so unfair to burden him mentally, when he was suffering so much physically as well.

I hadn't known how much he had heard on TV. He had heard it all. He just couldn't put the pieces together.

"Ben, you know how we explained to you that you got AIDS from the factor? There are a couple of other ways too. Drug addicts can get it, too, from dirty needles. But the most common way it's passed is through the gay community."

"That's what they talk about all the time on TV," Ben said. "About people who have AIDS being gay. What's *gay*, Dad?"

"Well, Ben, *gay* means people of the same sex who love each other. When people say *gay,* that's what they mean. Mostly they mean men."

Ben looked confused. Grant knew he had to say more and I could see him slowly, carefully choosing his words.

"You see, Ben, sometimes men love each other just the way a man and a woman love each other."

Grant went on to explain that our church teaches that that sort of love was reserved for a husband and wife.

"Is that why He's punishing them with AIDS?"

"No, Ben. I don't think so. God loves all his children, even those who do things he doesn't like."

"And He's not punishing me, either?"

"No, Ben. He is not punishing you. This is very, very important. Please don't ever think you did anything wrong, Ben. Because you didn't."

I reached over and hugged Ben. How I wished I could make this easier on him!

"You just got a germ, Benny," I told him. "That's all. When you get a cold, you don't think God's punishing you. Do you?"

That made sense to him.

"Heavenly Father loves you very, very much, Ben. That's why we're all praying to Him to help you get better. We all love you very much. And we don't want you to worry about this anymore, okay?

"Besides, I know one little boy in this household who is up way past his bedtime."

Ben went to bed relieved, satisfied with the explanation.

A few days later, Grant and I were getting ready to go out for our traditional Friday night "date." I was so glad it was Friday and so glad Grant was home. Our few hours alone on Friday nights were the fuel that allowed me to get through the rest of the week. Our dates gave us the strength we needed to endure and reminded us that we could get through this . . . together. The only escape we had from Ben's illness.

While I was dressing, the phone rang. It was my mother. She was calling Ben. They had such a special relationship, those two. And I was thrilled about it. Grandparents are special. They're the people who live in houses filled with good smells. People with cool, soft cheeks and wonderful laughs and lots of love. People who give you presents even when it's not your birthday.

I smiled as I listened to Ben's end of the conversation.

When he hung up, he told us he and Gramma had it all worked out. He was going to her house for a visit. After all, Beau and Aber had gotten to go to her house while he was in the hospital. Now it was his turn.

I didn't say anything. And seeing my hesitation, Grant told Ben we'd talk about it in the morning.

For now, it was Friday night.

"What should we do, go to a movie?" Grant asked.

We saw a lot of movies. Comedies, mostly. But there weren't enough of them around. So sometimes we'd just have dinner together. Being together, that's all that mattered. Alone.

"There's that little restaurant you've been wanting to try," Grant suggested.

We got an intimate table in a corner and it felt like the ultimate luxury to us. Candlelight. Real napkins. Each other.

Grant reached over and took my hand.

"Chris, you need a break," he said. "Look at you. You're so tired. Think of the baby, if not yourself. I think it's a great idea for Ben to go stay with your mom for a few days."

"But Grant, just getting Ben to eat, getting that medicine down his throat that he hates. Today he just wouldn't let me do it. He said his throat was better and he didn't need it anymore. What if something happens?"

"Nothing will happen. He'll be fine. And we can take Beau and Aber down to my parents at the beach for a few days with us. It'll be like old times. Besides, Chris, he wants to go. We're not the only people in his life."

I knew that. But ever since he'd been sick, I hadn't wanted to let him out of my sight. He needed me. And I needed him. I felt the way I had when he was still an infant. I just couldn't quite let him go. But he wasn't an infant. And Grant was right. Ben was my first child. But he was also my mother's first grandchild. I had to share him.

"Okay," I said.

We both opened the menus. He studied his for a moment, closed it, and leaned over and whispered to me.

"Now that that's settled," he said, "let's elope."

"What? Oh. Sorry, I'm pretty slow tonight. All right. Where shall we go?"

"I hear there's a plane leaving for Hawaii tonight."

"Ah. Turtle Bay."

"Let's leave now and send for our things."

"Sounds great."

We were enjoying our evening and our fantasy escape until the hostess seated two gay men at the table next to us and brought us back to reality.

At first we tried to ignore them. Then the men started to get affectionate with each other and I couldn't stand it anymore.

I know it was irrational. But everywhere I looked there was something to remind me of AIDS. Couldn't I just steal my little Friday night of pleasure? Was it too much to ask?

"Let's go," I said to Grant. We hurriedly paid our check and left.

I didn't blame them. Not those two men. I didn't even know their names. But I was angry. Angry that there was no relief. Angry that no matter where we went or what we did, Ben still had AIDS. That there was no part of this planet where we could go to escape. No hideaway. No vacation spot. Somewhere there must be a place without AIDS in it. We could talk about it. We could see it in our minds. We just couldn't reach it.

We took Ben up to Stanford for a checkup before he went off to visit my mother. And while Dr. Glader was examining Ben, Beau and Aber were tested for AIDS. They asked Grant and me to be tested too, as part of a national study.

Dr. Glader was pleased with Ben. He wrote in his report

that Ben was "clinically better" and he told us that Ben had
gained weight and his spirits were high.

Ben had told the doctor all about the new house we were
moving into and the new school he would be attending.

"There's no reason why Ben can't start school," the doctor
said.

The five of us sang all the way home in the van. Sometimes
we sang on trips just to make the time pass. But this time we
sang because we were happy. We sang because Ben was getting
better.

The next day Grant and I stopped by the school and told
the principal about Ben. She'd be happy to have him, she told
us.

School was going to start in less than a month and Ben
would be able to check off yet another thing on his list of
things to look forward to. He was ready to go to Gramma's.

Once again, my folks agreed to drive halfway up to
Carmel and we would drive halfway down to Los Angeles.
I was worried as we drove down about leaving Ben. But Ben
was so excited.

We dropped him off, and the whole way home I thought
what a good time Ben would have. He loved all her antiques
and curios. Her potpourri and candles. Her house was like a
curiosity shop to him—there was always something new to
play with. I could imagine him out in the workshop with
Grampa Ralph working away on some new wood project.
Ben loved working in the workshop. By the time we got
home, I made myself content knowing Ben was content.

As much as I would miss Ben, this was time that I needed. Time to devote to Beau and Aber and time to get ready for the move to our new house. We stayed busy all day until late that evening, when the phone rang.

"Chris," my mother's voice said. "I wanted you to know we made it safely."

"Good," I said. "How's Ben?"

"He's fine, but Chris . . . Ben's worried . . . where do I begin? Ben's afraid you'll . . ."

"What is it, Mom? What's wrong?"

"Nothing's wrong. He's asleep. I gave him a strawberry bubble bath, the kind I used to give you when you were little, and put him to bed. But there's something you need to know. Ben and I had a long talk tonight. We sat down at the dining-room table, and he just stroked that little wooden whale—you know, the one Ralph made that we keep on the coffee table and that he likes so much. And . . . well, Chris . . . Ben knows he's going to die and he's afraid you and Grant are going to be mad at him . . . he wanted me to call you."

"Mad at him? Mad at him for what?"

"He's afraid you'll be mad at him if he dies . . ."

My mother was crying off and on as she told me about the rest of their conversation.

"He asked me first if I would be mad at him if he died and went back to live with Heavenly Father, and I told him no. That of course I wouldn't, that I loved him, that he was the one who made me a Gramma. And then he said he didn't know about you and Grant, that maybe you would be mad because you'd had him so long now and you loved him so much."

"Did you tell him we wouldn't ever, ever be mad at him?"

"Yes, honey. That's exactly what I said."

My mom had always had a way of drawing people out. She had always been one of those people others go to for help. Even Ben . . .

I was glad she was there for him. I knew that Ben and I would have our time to talk too. But that time hadn't come. Not yet.

All I could think of right now was that I didn't want to be having this conversation. I could talk to the doctors about Ben's "prognosis." But then we were talking about a patient and AIDS. Now it was Mom I was talking to, and she was talking about Ben dying.

"He just needs a little reassurance," she said. "You know, that everything's okay."

"Yes, Mom. I'll talk to him. We have talked to him. But we didn't want to say too much about what the doctors had told us because we didn't want to scare him. And he's doing pretty well right now. We're still praying that . . ."

"I know, Chris, we are too. Thanks for letting Ben come. I know it's hard to let him go, but we'll take good care of him."

"Thanks for telling me, Mom."

"Good night, Chris. And don't worry about him. He's fine."

"Good night, Mom. I love you."

That weekend, Grant and I took off with Aber and Beau to the beach at San Clemente, where Grant's parents live. And for a long weekend, we were just a normal family again. We bought ice cream cones. We built sand castles. I worried about putting enough zinc ointment on Beau and Aber's noses again. Sunburn was the biggest worry I had at the beach. And it was nice.

Maybe if I hadn't seen Ben next to his little brothers with their freckles and red noses, I wouldn't have been so shocked by his appearance when we walked in the door at my mother's house to pick up Ben.

He was lying on the sofa, weak and listless and thinner by far than I had seen him. For the first time, the thought entered my mind: *Could this be it?*

He lifted his head to kiss Grant and me. And as weak as he was, he couldn't wait to tell Beau and Aber about his stay. The two of them, so healthy-looking, sat down on the couch next to Ben. They wanted to hear every detail.

I turned to go into the kitchen and Grant followed me. He put his arms around my shoulders. He was as shocked as I was to see Ben this way. How could it have happened so fast? My mother could see how upset we both were when she came into the room.

"Mom, he looks . . . really bad. He's so pale."

"It's just been for the last three days. He did great the first few days he was here. But he just couldn't eat. He couldn't keep anything down. And he really tried. He wanted to eat. I didn't know what else to do."

Even as she spoke, I caught sight of the five different kinds of soup cans opened, lined up on the kitchen counter. It looked like my kitchen when I was trying everything I knew to find something, anything Ben could stomach. I knew how hard she had tried. And I knew the frustration she felt.

"What are we going to do, Mom?"

She put her arms around me and hugged me the way she used to when I was little.

Then Ben came in and said he and Grampa wanted to show me something outside.

We went out the back door to the picnic table. Ralph had worked at a soda fountain when he was young where the customers were encouraged to carve their initials in the counter. Ralph was a master craftsman who had worked with wood his whole life. He was taken with the soda fountain idea and had decided to carry out the tradition with the family picnic table.

Every time grandchildren came over, they got to carve something in it with a little electric penknife. Ben had made a new contribution. I didn't know whether to laugh or cry when I saw it. It was a perfectly drawn, almost life-size hamburger. Complete with sesame seeds and lettuce.

"He worked real hard on it," Ralph said. "Just practiced and practiced on a piece of wood first. You know, he'd make a real fine artist someday."

"Thanks, Ralph," I said, kissing him on the cheek. "You mean a lot to Ben."

I started picking up Ben's things while Grant carried Ben

to the van. How hard this must be for my mother. It wasn't just her grandchild she was watching suffer so. It was her child too. It was me. I loved her so much. Whenever I really needed her, she was always there.

That trip became a touchstone for Ben in the long, difficult months that followed. He often retold little stories about things that had happened on the strawberry-bubble-bath trip. That was how it became known in our family. About going to a movie with his cousins Brett and Joey and laughing and spilling popcorn all over everyone. About how he and Grampa made two birdhouses—one for Gramma and one for me. About a dozen things that didn't mean much except that they turned the light on in his eyes.

On the way home, Ben asked if we could go up to the hospital. He knew how sick he was. He didn't say much to the doctors who examined him when we checked in. He weighed thirty-four pounds, less than his three-year-old brother. He held his arm out for the nurse who came to hook him up to the now-familiar IV. He knew he had to be here now.

That night, after Grant and the boys had left to go back to Carmel, I sat with Ben on the edge of the bed in his old room and watched as he tried to eat a little dinner.

I understood it now. Ben wasn't really closer to dying, and he wouldn't be further away from death when he came home, no matter how much care we gave him. The fact was we'd bring him back here where they could pump him up, and for a couple weeks he would feel better, look better.

But Ben never pretended he was getting better. We were

the ones who pretended. That was the only way we had gotten through this summer. It was human. It was just normal. We were normal, Grant and Beau and Aber and I. We'd gotten the AIDS test results back. Those too were normal. It was normal for Aber to keep asking if Ben was better. It was normal for us to pray for miracles.

We had sunburns and parking tickets and all the other kinds of things normal people have. Only we weren't normal really. Because Ben was dying. And he was afraid. Not afraid of dying. That's not what he had said. Afraid that we would be mad at him for dying. That's what he had told my mother.

Did he . . . could he possibly believe that somehow he would be letting us down? That what worried him most was hurting us? How could I tell him?

"I missed you when you were gone, Ben," I said. "I know why you wanted to go. And it was all right with me. You know I could never be mad at you for just going on a trip, don't you? Not even if it lasted for a long, long time. I would only be sad that we weren't together, and I'd miss you a lot."

Ben nodded and handed me his tray. He was tired.

"I missed you too, Mom," he said. He gave me a big hug and then settled back into bed.

"I love you to pieces."

I could hear the sounds of the hospital settling in for the night, the dinner trays being rolled down the corridors, the squeaky sound of nurses' rubber soles on the floor.

I knew there was more I was supposed to say. But I couldn't say it. Not tonight.

4

"Help Me, Mom"

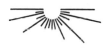

IT WAS HARDER than ever to leave Ben the next day. But I had no choice. I had to go home and pack. I kissed him good-bye about noon. And about the same time in Carmel, Grant put away his tools and headed up to the hospital. We crossed somewhere along the freeway. And while he was greeting Ben, I was unlocking our door to start packing.

It was already Thursday, and we had to be out of our duplex apartment on Saturday. Two more days, I told myself, and things would be better. We would be living in our own house. Ben would have his very own room, and something else on his list would come true. We could all get a fresh start.

I didn't realize how much packing there was to do. It was such a small place, after all. And Grant had already done some of it while I was gone. But by dinnertime, when I picked up the boys at a friend's house, where Grant had left them that morning, I realized I had hardly made any progress at all. I couldn't seem to concentrate. Part of me was still back in that hospital room with Ben.

I remember stumbling around bleary-eyed, looking for the masking tape about midnight. And I had one of those household things in my hand that doesn't belong anywhere, I don't know what, a yardstick or an extension cord. So I went from room to room trying to find the right box for it, hoping to find the tape too. But all I saw were other things there were no boxes for.

Everywhere I looked there were opened drawers and cupboards, all of them still half full. And all over the floors there were cardboard boxes, still half empty. I wondered how I would get through it.

For the first time in my life, I'm not going to be able to do something I absolutely have to do. I'm not going to be able to pack this house up to be ready to move out the day after tomorrow. I can't pack a simple cardboard box. And I don't have the energy or the willpower to try to figure it out.

I've been running on emergency fuel ever since Ben got sick, and the emergency's still on but my energy has run out. Just like that. Gone. It's finally happened. I can't cope anymore. I can't.

I just collapsed on the sofa and shut my eyes.

Sleep. All I wanted was to sleep. For days and days. For weeks maybe. And then I'd wake up and Ben would be cured, and we would be living in our new house, and I wouldn't have to remember where I put the masking tape.

It was so tempting.

Then another voice told me I couldn't do that. I couldn't give up. Not me, Chris, who always did everything she had to do.

I just sat there, seven months pregnant, stupefied by confusion and exhaustion. I didn't know how to do what I had to do. And I didn't know how not to. I was too overwhelmed to move in either direction.

I'm not sure how long I sat there. Maybe fifteen minutes. Maybe more. Finally I reached for the phone and dialed.

"Mom," I said in a voice that sounded so pathetic I hardly recognized it. "I don't know what to do."

I didn't care how desperate I sounded, or how exhausted. I had no resources left and nowhere else to turn. Only my mother would know what to do. My mother the organizer.

"Mom . . . help me. I can't think anymore. Everything's all, all . . . And I don't know how to get it . . . And I just can't think anymore. I just want you to tell me what to do. Tell me exactly what to do so I can write it down and do it."

I unburdened myself of all the things ahead of me. The packing, the cleaning at the new house, the meals for the boys, the calls to Ben, a doctor's appointment the next day.

"Slow down, honey," she said. "Get your notebook and your pen and I'm going to tell you three things to put at the top of your list. Write these down. Okay? Grant. The boys. And yourself. Just those three. And when you worry about the other things, look at that list and take care of those things first. Because they count. The other things don't count. You just have to do them."

Of course. That sounded so clear. But somehow all the important things had gotten jumbled up in my mind with all the little things. And the little things always had to get done now, while the things that mattered got put off. Like now. When did I have time to spend with Grant? I hadn't even seen him all day.

"But Mom, we've got to be out of here by Saturday and

we have people coming over to help us move into the new house."

"Would you like me to come up and help?"

"I'd rather save your visit for another time, Mom. I don't want to waste it on this."

My mother paused.

"Okay, I'll give you a list of things to do and by Saturday you'll have them done, and then you'll reward yourself by doing something that's one of those three things up there that's important, all right?"

"All right."

"Okay. Now first I want you to go to sleep and wake up in the morning fresh. And when you get up . . ."

I put her list by my bed that night, and when I got up in the morning, I followed it right down the line like a robot. I didn't want to even let myself think. Get up. Get dressed. Make the bed so you have someplace neat to return to. Make breakfast . . . Pack the bedroom, then the bathroom . . .

That night, after the boxes were all packed, I took Beau and Aber over to the new house so I could clean the kitchen there. It was dark, a little spooky in the empty house, as I made a bed for the boys on the carpet in the living room.

I scrubbed the kitchen for an hour or more. I actually enjoyed the cleaning because I had something to show for it when I was done. Nothing I did anymore seemed to make much of a difference.

And when my swollen ankles told me I had to stop, I went

in and sat by Beau and Aber for just a minute before loading them into the van and going back home.

Moving had always been a bittersweet time for me, a mix of leaving something behind and starting something new. Here we were, leaving behind a small apartment we had outgrown, and moving into our first house, the kind of place Grant and I had been talking about ever since we had been engaged. Not a mansion or a brand-new split-level. A homey little place we could work on and remodel and turn into something that reflected our family. Someplace warm, with a special spot in the kitchen to tack up drawings the boys would bring home from school.

I watched Beau and Aber as they slept.

What went through their minds when they looked at Ben? Did they know he was dying? Did Beau understand, really understand, that AIDS meant he might not have a big brother around anymore? What about Abraham? What could a three-year-old possibly understand of dying?

What would life be like in this place for Beau and Aber? For Ben? What would the days be like that he would spend in his room down the hall? How long—how many weeks, how many months, how many years—would he have to live in this house with us?

I couldn't think about that now. I was too exhausted to think about anything. I had to get home.

Grant came in from the hospital late that night. The next day was moving day.

It wasn't much after 7 A.M. when we heard the toot of the

Laceys' old Volvo wagon. Joe was a retired Army lieutenant colonel from our church; Mary, a retired teacher. They had often taken care of Beau and Aber while I was at the hospital.

I went out on the front lawn to greet them. But it wasn't just Joe and Mary. There were the Karchners, too, and the Smiths. And as I watched, a whole line of trucks and cars turned the corner one by one, and drove down our little street like a parade. A whole parade of people coming to help. Members of our church, good close friends. The teenaged girls I'd taught. And the men from Grant's church group. People with good hearts who had asked us every Sunday if there was anything they could do. People I had always said no to because I didn't even know where to begin, and because I wasn't used to needing help.

Now, they had all found something they could do. The men started hauling out furniture and boxes. The women helped me finish cleaning. And one of my former students watched Beau and Aber.

By late afternoon, I couldn't believe my eyes. We were moved in. Our house was clean. There was shelf paper in the cupboard. The freezer was full of casseroles and desserts and everything we would need for a week. And the old maple bedstead and dresser that had belonged to Grampa Oyler when he was a boy had at last been taken down from the attic and were sitting in Ben's new room waiting for him to come home.

Grant and I were tired but excited. I remember we were leaning against the living-room wall surveying our work when we both just slid down and sat next to each other on the floor.

"How would it look to build in some bookcases over there on either side of the fireplace?" I asked.

"Maybe we should expand the kitchen and put on a second story," Grant said. "We could use the space once Chelsea arrives."

I leaned over and kissed him.

"You know the only thing I really want?"

"Me?" he asked, joking.

"Besides you. A round kitchen table. It's cozier than a square one, somehow. You can see everybody talk. It's more like a family circle."

Grant and I had begun to dream again, to dream dreams that had a chance of coming true. We had begun to talk about the future as if it held something to look forward to. I guess even grown-ups need lists of things to look forward to sometimes.

We drove up to get Ben two days later.

He was feeling much better again, and when we got home, he ran straight down to his new room to check it out.

"Dad! Mom! It's great!" he shouted. "Grampa's furniture!"

I helped Ben put up his Star Wars poster and hang his wooden dinosaurs and his model airplanes from the ceiling and set up the family computer we had decided to put in Ben's room.

Except for the medicine in the closet, the room began to look like Ben. Our Ben.

Just as I was turning down Ben's sheets, Beau and Aber came tearing down the hall and leaped into Ben's bed, where Ben promptly joined them. I turned around to see Grant come stalking into the room in his scariest big-bear walk and his fiercest big-bear growl. I laughed.

Leave it to Grant. I just loved this part of him, this part that was still such a little boy. He gave me the quickest unbearlike little grin and then jumped into bed in the middle of his sons.

"Once upon a time . . . there was the hugest, scariest black bear in the woods and he had these giant fangs and these mean, beady little eyes. And one day, he came tromping out of the woods. Tromp, tromp, tromp . . ."

Grant stopped to growl again. He really had the hungry-bear growl down.

"And what do you think he saw? Three little boys playing in their brand-new backyard. That's what he saw. And you know what their names were?"

"Ben!" said Ben.

"Beau!" said Beau.

"And Aber!" said Aber.

I leaned against the doorway for a while and listened. Grant's big booming bear voice mixed with the boys' excited little ones.

Their voices were turning this unfamiliar new house into a home, an Oyler home. Grant's father had told him this story when he was a boy, just as I'm sure he'd heard it from his father when he was small.

I went back to our room and undressed for bed. I was exhausted. But I was happy too, happier than I had been in months. I could go to sleep secure in the knowledge that the bravest little boy of the evening would growl back at the bear, and stick his arm way, way down inside the bear's throat, grab the bear by the tail and turn him inside out . . . and save the day.

And that everybody, at least in the story, would live happily ever after.

We spent the next week unpacking boxes, building Darcy a fence in the backyard, and searching out a place where we could plant a garden someday. All of us working together. The house still needed a lot of work, but what was truly important was those three things my mother had told me in my moment of despair. And I had them all: my husband, my children—and my sanity.

The day before school was supposed to start, Grant and I went down to talk to the principal of Carmel River School. We wanted to explain to her that Ben probably wouldn't be able to go full time, at least at first. But he would be able to go a couple hours a day and meet his new classmates. That was what mattered the most to him now. He had been in and out of the hospital so often that he had gone almost all summer without any friends around. And now he was starting at a new school.

"There may be a . . . delay," she told us. "Not with Beau, of course. Just with Ben."

"A delay? What delay? We talked to you about this a few

weeks ago and there was no problem," I said. I felt tense. They couldn't do this to Ben now. Not after we had checked and they had said it would be okay. Why hadn't somebody told us? Didn't they understand Ben had been looking forward to this all summer long?

"Mrs. Oyler, surely you've noticed that we've had a school board election. We have a new board now. A new superintendent. Maybe you'd better take it up with him."

Grant and I couldn't believe our ears. We knew there had been a boy in New York with AIDS who couldn't go to school because parents were so terrified their kids would get it. That was all over the evening news every night. But we'd talked to the school in advance to make sure it was okay. It was all settled. At least, as far as we knew, it *had* been all settled.

"How soon can we talk to the new superintendent and get this straightened out?" Grant asked.

"I'll call, but I know he's going to be busy, since tomorrow is the first day of school," she said. We were well aware of that. It was supposed to be Ben's first day too.

We were given an appointment for Thursday—two days after school started. All we could tell Ben was that he would have to wait a couple of days to start school. He was disappointed, but it was going to be only two more days.

"We've run into a little problem," Dr. Robert Infelice, the superintendent, said as we sat down in his office. "You see, we have some parents who are very much against Ben's going to school and we need to ease into this. The board could vote, and maybe by November . . ."

"Well, what can we do? Could we do something to help inform people about AIDS? Some . . . some community meetings maybe?" I asked.

"Well, first we have to work with the staff and the teachers . . . maybe by November . . ."

November? That was two more months. Couldn't they understand what two months meant to Ben?

"But Ben's ready to go to school now. He's been looking forward to this all summer. You just don't know what this means to him."

"It means a lot to other parents, too. And to our board. A lot of things are at stake here."

"But those children can't catch AIDS from Ben. Studies have shown it. If you could get AIDS from Ben, don't you think his little brothers would have it by now, or me or my husband?"

"I understand. It must be very difficult for you. But think of your son, Mrs. Oyler. Wouldn't a home tutor be a little more suitable? I'm sure he's not really up to spending all day long in a classroom, is he?

"He's very susceptible to infection, isn't he? This is for his own protection. Kids can be . . . well, cruel to other children who have special needs. We wouldn't want him to attend school in a hostile environment. And I'm afraid that's what it would be."

How did he know what was right for Ben?

"There's more to school than education, Dr. Infelice," Grant said. "There's being around other children. There's making friends and learning to get along with other people. The kids could learn a lot from Ben, too."

The board's mind was made up, he said. They had a legal obligation to educate Ben and they would. Only on their terms. They would give him a home tutor when he was up to it. And they would hold community hearings to educate the public about AIDS. Then the board would vote again and we'd see.

That was all.

On our way home, Grant and I talked about it. I couldn't understand why we hadn't been consulted or even considered in this decision. Why had it been kept so hush-hush? Then just dumped on us? And we were supposed to just go along with it and be content. I had a right to be mad about this. It was unfair! So silly! Their minds were made up already, and the only way to fight it would be to go public. Like the family of the little boy in New York. But did we really want to do that? To subject ourselves to the public scrutiny of a lawsuit? Of television cameras on our front lawn? What would all that publicity do to Ben? Was that the way we wanted to spend our energy? No. What energy we had left we wanted to put into quality time with Ben.

Still, we weren't ready to give up. Not this easily. We'd just have to fight on the school board's terms. But how would we tell Ben he couldn't go to school? What else would he have to look forward to now? The only other thing I could think of was Cub Scouts. Ben already had his uniform. I called the new Cub Scout leader to see if Ben was still welcome there. She said she'd be delighted to have Ben at their first meeting later that week.

"Ben, look, it's almost ready," I said that afternoon, holding up his uniform with the patches sewn on.

"That's great, Mom," he said.

"Ben, come here, there's something I want to talk to you about, okay?" I said, patting the sofa next to me.

He came over and held up his new uniform.

"Very handsome," I said. "But Ben, I've got some bad news for you."

He looked at me.

"What, Mom?"

"It's school, Ben. You can't start tomorrow."

I could see the tears rise in his eyes.

"Why not?"

"Remember how we talked about AIDS being a little scary because it's so new? Well, it's kind of scary to other people too. They don't understand it yet. So the people who run the school are going to try to teach other people about it before you go. It may take a couple months. Maybe even a little longer. But in the meantime they're going to give you a teacher to come here and help you keep up."

"You mean Beau can go and I can't?"

I nodded. What could I say? That was exactly it.

"Ben, I'm sorry. Dad and I want you to know that we don't like this at all."

"But I won't get to meet any of the new kids."

"We're going to keep trying to get you back in school as soon as we can. For now, Ben, we'll have to find other ways to meet new friends. There's the Cub Scout meeting next week. Right?"

He just thought for a while and I wondered what was going on inside his little head.

"I was really looking forward to school. But don't worry, Mom. It's okay. But could I ride my bike to school with Beau anyway? He's pretty little, Mom. Just a first-grader. He needs somebody like me to help him."

It was Ben who had taught Beau to ride a two-wheeler.

"Are you sure you're up to it?"

"It's downhill all the way, Mom."

"Most of the way, you mean. But I guess it'll be all right. Beau is pretty little still. But please be careful and stay together."

I hugged Ben. Sometimes he amazed me. He was more concerned about Beau than he was about himself. Ben asked so little and he never complained. What mattered most to him was the people he loved. I thought to myself that children are so forgiving.

He and Beau took off early the next morning. Ben put on his new school clothes with his suspenders. And they were both so excited, taking off on this little adventure of theirs. It had been a while since Ben had ridden a bike.

"Help Me, Mom"

I kissed them good-bye and waited.

The phone rang about thirty minutes later. It was Ben's voice. He was too weak to ride home. Could I come get him?

I found Ben waiting out in front of the school. The first thing he did was apologize for having gone into the school when he wasn't supposed to. That made me angrier the more I thought about it. Here was an eight-year-old apologizing for going to school.

As we drove home with the bike in the back of the van, Ben couldn't wait to tell me about it.

"We had a great time going down the hill, Mom," he said. "You shoulda seen us. We were just tearin' down there, Beau 'n' me."

"And you helped Beau get to school all right?"

"Sure, Mom. I did. He sure has a nice teacher. Could I go look around his class sometime . . . maybe after school? His teacher said it would be okay."

He was quiet the rest of the way home. Later that morning he came into the kitchen to see me.

"Mom, can you put an ad in the paper for me?"

"What for, Ben?"

"I want to sell my bike."

I think that was the moment I realized how much Ben was changing. Things like bicycles and break dancing and school didn't matter so much to Ben anymore. His mind, indeed his soul, was working toward something greater.

Grant and I were the ones who had held on to those hopes of tomorrow. That Ben would break dance again. That Ben would ride his bike again. That Ben would feel good and strong again. Those elusive tomorrows.

But four months of tomorrows had come and gone. And Ben wasn't really getting better. The hospital could pump him up and make him stronger for a few days, but the tomorrow Grant and I dreamed of wasn't going to come. Ben knew that even if we didn't.

It was like the stories you hear about people who get an incredible surge of power and energy in an emergency. Power they never knew they had. Ben had that. Deep inside him there was a source that helped him understand and accept and not be afraid. We were the ones who kept being afraid. Afraid of an ending. But Ben could see a beginning—a beginning that would take him away from us but to a place we had taught him not to fear.

As strong as our faith was, I realize now, it was still pretty theoretical. We had never had to come face to face with it the way Ben had to now.

We had prepared our minds and our souls. But we hadn't prepared our emotions. How could we? There was no way that living could prepare you for dying. Not really.

No matter how strong our faith, when it came right down to it, we were just two young parents who didn't want their son to die.

As the school year began and it became known that there was a boy in the school district with AIDS, Ben's story was on television every night and in the newspapers every morning. He was the anonymous little boy with AIDS. His name was never mentioned, because we decided not to fight it publicly. Only our family, a few friends, and some people at school knew it was Ben. So Ben became the seventy-seventh hemophiliac in the United States to be diagnosed as having AIDS, the third-grader with AIDS from River School.

There were public hearings, and local doctors testified that no family member of any AIDS victim had ever been found to have AIDS. Not one. But the statistics didn't matter. The other parents' minds were made up. They were scared. And nothing the doctors said, nothing health agencies said, and nothing the Hemophilia Foundation said made any difference.

AIDS, or rather the fear of AIDS, had invaded our little community.

I was sitting at the car wash one day when the lady next to me brought up the subject. "Don't you think it's terrible, that family who wants their son with AIDS to go to school?" I didn't reply.

She continued. "I certainly wouldn't want any child of mine in school with him."

"Well, if you really look into it there's no way your child could be in any danger. AIDS can't be transmitted through casual contact . . . like at school."

"They don't know that for sure."

My car came up and I gladly said good-bye to the lady. She had no idea she had been talking to the mother of the child she thought was so dangerous. It was like being in a goldfish bowl, only people couldn't see our faces. They wanted to stare at us but they didn't know where to look. They wanted to ostracize us but they didn't know how to find us.

Though we managed to keep the television people away from Ben, it was much harder to keep Ben away from television. When he saw the first broadcast about himself, he was excited to be a celebrity. Pretty soon that wore off. "I'd rather just go to school like everybody else," he said.

He couldn't go to school. But he did go to his Cub Scout meeting. The troop leader kissed him and waved to me as I dropped him off. And when I picked him up, he came out with a bunch of colorful balloons made out of construction paper. He had written his name in glue and then covered it with glitter. There it was in shining script: "Ben Oyler."

But as September wore on, Ben grew weaker. The saddest part of our fight with the school district was that Ben couldn't have gone to school anyway. He wasn't even up to having a tutor. There were days when he couldn't get out of bed, whole days when he couldn't keep any food or medicine down. He wasn't even up to playing with Beau and Aber.

I think Beau was hit the hardest by the controversy surrounding Ben. Harder, even, than Ben himself. Beau had always been so proud of being Ben Oyler's brother. And now he was at a brand-new school where the only thing his classmates knew about him was that he was the brother of the boy with AIDS.

I talked with his teacher, who was wonderful. She protected him from the cameras and called me from time to time that year to let me know how he was doing.

"Help Me, Mom"

The first time she called was just the second week of school. Beau couldn't seem to concentrate, she said. He couldn't seem to finish any work. He'd start and then just kind of stare off into space. I'd noticed the same thing at home. I had talked to him. But I didn't know how to help him. I couldn't change the cause of the problem. His teacher and I decided it was best not to push him for now. I made a mental note to ask Judie Lea about counseling the next time we went up to the hospital.

I was hanging Ben's sheets out on the line one day to make them smell fresh for him when Beau came running out. Beau was as different from Ben as night from day. Whereas Ben was thoughtful, sometimes quiet, Beau was straightforward.

"Mom, Ben's no fun anymore," he told me. "He kicked me 'n' Aber out of his room and he told us to stay out. He never wants to do anything anymore."

I put the laundry aside and sat down on the grass with Beau.

"Ben's just sick, Beau, that's all."

"Ben's always sick, Mom."

"Remember when you were sick with the flu? You didn't feel like doing anything, did you? You didn't want Ben and Aber jumping on your bed or making noise or asking you to run outside and play because you just felt bad inside."

Beau stared at the grass. He remembered.

"Well, Beau, that's what Ben feels like all the time now. All day long and all night too. It hurts him a lot that he can't play with you the same way anymore. It's frustrating, isn't it?"

"I want the old Ben back, Mom. I miss him . . . the way he used to be. When will Ben be fun again, Mom?"

"I don't know, Beau. Ben may be sick for a long, long time. He may never feel like the old Ben again. But he wants you and Aber to play with him more than he ever did before. Only you have to play different games with him now. Quiet games. Games where you don't have to run. And you have to be patient with him. Just the way he had to be patient with you when you were little. Do you think you can do that?"

Beau was looking down but I could see tears start to roll off his nose. I leaned forward and let him cry in my arms for a minute.

"I still wanna play with Ben, Mom. But I don't think Ben wants to play with me . . . Mom, I don't think Ben likes me anymore."

"Oh, Beau! Ben loves you! Ben loves you very, very much. And don't you ever forget that, okay?"

"Okay."

Beau said he understood. I wasn't sure. I left our little talk wondering, feeling as though something was unresolved, incomplete.

The next morning Ben got out of the shower, as he did every day now, shivering and unsteady on his feet. This time, he happened to have his back to me. And I was shocked, all of a sudden, to see how thin he was. I could count every rib. His skin just hung loose and lifeless over the bones underneath. And when he walked, the cheeks of his little bottom lapped against the back of his thighs. They were only skin, with no flesh underneath.

It took my breath away to see him. When had Ben turned into a skeleton? Why hadn't I realized it earlier? Had I wanted so much for him to be better that I hadn't noticed how terribly, terribly ill he really was? Why, there was no flesh left on him. None at all. I could see each vertebra in his back. And his legs were so thin his knees seemed as big as baseballs. He was quite literally just skin and bones.

I took a big towel and wrapped it around him. I wanted to warm him, to cover him, to hold him and tell him I loved him.

I was so scared.

We had to do something. But I didn't know what. I had tried and tried to get him to eat. When he wouldn't eat at mealtimes, we'd go down the list of all his favorite foods. But all the homemade grilled cheese sandwiches and sprints across town to get tacos weren't making any difference, because he couldn't keep them down.

That night after the boys were in bed, I was sitting in the living room waiting for Grant to come home. He had been working such long hours, trying to make up for time he'd missed the week before.

I turned on the television set. On the screen was a special about famine in Ethiopia. The camera kept focusing on the children. Children with huge eyes and hollow cheeks who were just waiting to die.

That's what Ben looks like, I thought.

Ben is dying of starvation. Only we're not living in Africa. This is America. My cupboards are full of food. And I can't stop him from starving.

I was sobbing by the time Grant came in.

"Chris," he said gently. "Why don't you shut it off if it bothers you that much?"

"It's not the show . . . it's Ben. Look at those children. Ben looks just like them. Exactly like them . . ."

"C'mon, Chris . . . it's not that bad."

"Grant, he's starving to death!"

Grant just looked down. I could see him fighting back the tears, telling himself that he had to be strong, for both of us. He put his arms around me.

"This is just one of those dark days. We've got to have faith he'll get better. We've just got to trust that he'll pull through this. He will. I just know it."

"Grant, I want a miracle as much as you do . . . but you're not here during the day. You're not trying to force that medicine down his throat. I am. And it's not working. It's just not working at all. Look at him tomorrow morning when he gets out of the shower.

"Grant, we have got to do something. Something quick. Otherwise we're going to lose Ben. I won't stand by and watch my child starve to death. I won't."

5

Our First Miracle

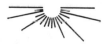

I KNEW THERE WAS NO QUICK ANSWER for Ben. But I couldn't get it out of my mind that somewhere, just beyond the horizon, there was another approach we could try. A new treatment soon to be written up in a medical journal. A new drug still being tested in a laboratory somewhere, or an unusual combination of vitamins that had brought success in Switzerland maybe, or France.

Because if we didn't find an alternative treatment, I didn't think Ben would make it until Christmas. And I was afraid he'd never get to see his baby brother or sister.

I was eight months pregnant already; the baby was due in early November. Somehow, through all the months of pain and uncertainty, the miracle of life was proceeding inside me as if nothing had changed. Even as my first-born son was dying, a new child inside me was preparing to be born. A child I had barely had time to think about. A child who did not yet have a nursery, nor even a name.

Ben had a very special sort of bond with the baby already. "How's the baby doing today, Mom?" he'd often ask me in the morning. Then, if the baby was up and kicking, I'd let him feel the little elbows and knees as they wriggled around inside me.

The baby had been on Ben's list of things to look forward

to back in May. But then, it was really a little brother he had in mind, a boy who would one day round out a team. Now it was a baby he was looking forward to, a baby he would finally be able to see and hold and love.

Only now I was afraid he would never get the chance.

I called Judie Lea to arrange to take Ben back up to the hospital, and to set aside a time to talk with the doctors.

When we arrived, the nurses had to try vein after vein before they could finally insert the IV that would alleviate Ben's dehydration. His veins were so weak now they kept collapsing.

It wasn't until the day after our arrival that I found a source of hope, in the form of a little boy walking down the hall with a Hickman catheter.

We had heard about the Hickman for the first time from, of all people, Beau. During one of Ben's early stays at the hospital, Beau had played with a little boy who had leukemia. That boy's name was Ben too. And he had a small rubber tube coming out of his chest. He had shown it to Beau and told him that that was how he ate, that they gave him nourishment through that tube. And Beau had pointed it out to us.

We asked about it when we got back up to the hospital.

"It's called a Hickman catheter," Judie Lea told Grant and me. "We were talking about it ourselves. I know the doctors planned to mention it to you. They think it might give Ben the nutritional buffer he needs right now."

Our appointment with the doctors was the following day. They told us then that there was no point in continuing the experimental Canadian antibiotic upon which we had based our hopes that summer. I wasn't surprised. It wasn't working. But giving up on that medicine meant giving up. And giving up was unthinkable.

The more we heard about the Hickman catheter, the more it seemed like the answer to our prayers. It wasn't a promise that Ben would live, for the doctors were very careful to remind us that this was not a cure. But with the catheter, Ben at least would not die of starvation.

The catheter was a small rubber tube that would be inserted surgically into a large vein in Ben's upper chest. And through that tubing he would get all his medicine and a personalized formula of liquid food. The Hickman wouldn't take away the AIDS, but it would make it much easier for him to live with it.

"You mean I won't be hungry anymore?" Ben asked in absolute astonishment when he first heard about the Hickman.

"And they won't have to stick you anymore, either," Grant said. "No more pokes. They'll put all your medicine through the Hickman."

"All right!"

"We want this to be your decision, Ben," I said. "Every night we'll have to hook you up to this machine that pumps your nourishment and medicine in. That means you can't ever just say you don't want to do it, because you won't have a choice. You'll be free all day. But at night, every night for twelve hours, you'll have to get hooked up."

Ben thought about it for all of three seconds.

"But there won't be any more shots? You promise?"

"I promise. No more shots. No more IVs."

"That's great, Mom. When can I get it?"

We couldn't schedule the operation until October. It was the first date available. But as soon as we got home, Grant and I found we wanted some reassurance that this was the right step to take, medically. The reality was that if we went ahead with the Hickman, Ben would be literally living on a machine for the rest of his life.

So, Grant asked the bishop of our church, Dr. Rasband, and his wife, Esther, over one night. Jim Rasband was a medical doctor as well as the leader of our congregation in Carmel. When they arrived, Grant brought them up to date on Ben's condition.

"We don't see how he can last much longer. He's just wasting away," Grant said. "And this Hickman seems like the only answer."

"Maybe," Dr. Rasband said. "But maybe it could also just prolong Ben's suffering. Have you thought about that? Is that what you want to do?"

I watched Grant's face. This was very hard on him. I had spent more time with Ben than he had. I had seen on an hourly basis how his little body was slowly giving in to this awful disease. It wasn't that I had accepted the fact that Ben was going to die. But by September, I believe I had accepted the fact that I would have to accept it someday. And Grant hadn't.

I answered for both of us.

"He's suffering now," I said. "If he doesn't have the Hickman, he's going to starve to death. And I just can't stand by and let him. Not when there's something we can finally do for him. I just can't."

The bishop's wife spoke quietly. She had two boys of her own. "Neither could I," she said quietly.

We decided to go ahead with the surgery.

But Dr. Rasband had asked us questions that we were already wrestling with ourselves. Questions I can formulate far more clearly now, looking back on that difficult year, than I could while we were actually living through it.

Were we doing this for Ben or for ourselves? Were we trying to keep Ben alive because we couldn't face his death? Because even if Ben was ready, we were not? And, if we weren't ready now, how in the world could there ever come a time when we would be?

After all, how could a parent give up on the fight for a child's life?

❧   ❧   ❧

Ben had the operation on October 2.

I remember the date because the surgery was the first subject Ben wrote about in his journal. The journal was a little present from some children who would have been in his class at school.

He wrote:

Wednesday afternoon I was taken in a ambulance to Stanford Hospital. Then I was taken upsairs in a elevator to the recoveyroom aftr a little while a doctor came in and gave me some stuff to make me go to sleep that I was rolled into the operating room and then I woke up in my room in childrens Hospital safe and sond.

At the bottom, he drew a picture of a large heart that had a little tube sticking out of it. Over the heart he pasted a sticker that was one of many that had come with his journal. "Good news!" it said.

And that Hickman was good news.

It gave us a glimpse of Ben once again, the way he had been before he got sick. We would be spared that awful feeling I'm sure many people feel when a member of their family is wrenched from them abruptly or sent spinning into a permanent downward spiral. Then family members find themselves living afterward not only with grief but with regrets.

Ben turned around after that operation and started to come back to us the first day after the surgery.

As soon as the liquid food could be pumped into his body to nourish him, he began to brighten and seem more alert. He was fascinated by the new tube coming out of his chest. He paid attention to every minute detail of the intricate procedures the nurses followed when cleaning it and hooking him up for the night to the pumps that would send the liquid food into his body. And if a nurse happened to deviate ever so slightly from a procedure, he would point out her error with unfailing accuracy.

Our First Miracle

The doctors had said it would take three to five weeks to balance Ben's nutritional needs and regulate the Hickman. So, the hospital became our home, Ben's and mine, for most of October. During that time, I would learn the procedures of caring for the Hickman and medicating Ben. And, when Grant was able, he would drive up after work and learn as well, and then drive home by midnight.

Beau and Aber went to stay once again with my mother and Ralph. And Ben and I settled in by ourselves, with Grant coming up whenever he could get away from work. He brought up my sewing machine, and the computer video games, and a VCR to rent movies, and a radio. While Ben listened to Michael Jackson and brushed up on the arm movements for his break dancing, I started on Ben's Halloween costume.

He wanted to be a Ninja warrior. Ninja warriors were popular that year. I didn't know much about them, except that they wore black silk karate-type suits and they used as weapons metal throwing stars that looked like circular saw blades. But to Ben they were as exciting as Star Wars characters had been the year before. He spent hours designing his costume. And when he was done, he gave me drawings of both front and back so I could make it exactly right, with a pouch in the back for the throwing stars. He even went to the fabric store with me for a couple of hours one day so he could pick out the right fabric.

When I finished the costume, Ben was so thrilled he tried it on and showed all the nurses. And one of them—Betsy was her name—was undoubtedly the only nurse in America who owned a genuine Ninja warrior throwing star with real Japanese writing on it. The next day, she brought it in and gave it to Ben. Her gift became a source of immense pride to Ben.

My mother took care of getting costumes for Beau and Aber. As the days passed, I began embroidering Christmas presents.

Occasionally, as I sewed, the baby inside me would get hiccups. And I would go over to Ben's bed and let him feel my stomach hiccuping. Ben would laugh, and I noticed he was getting his dimples back.

He loved this child, even before it was born. Sometimes I felt as if he were urging it on toward birth, coaxing it to come out into the world so the two of them would have more time with each other. He told me how lucky Aber would be to find out what it was like to be a big brother, a role he truly enjoyed himself. And how lucky we all would be to have a new baby just in time for Christmas.

I was almost nine months pregnant. My ankles were swollen all the time. Terrible-looking varicose veins had appeared on my legs. Each time before when I had been pregnant, these physical problems had been little more than a nuisance to me. They hadn't mattered at all, compared with the excitement of the child I was about to meet.

But now, it was as if Ben had taken on the job of being excited. I couldn't find it in me. I had been excited when I found out I was pregnant. But that was before Ben had gotten sick.

Since then, my emotions had been stretched out so far that they had simply stretched out, like an old piece of elastic. And they wouldn't stretch back. I wanted to feel excited about this baby, the way I had been with my other three. I kept hoping the excitement would come, but for now all I could think of was the work ahead of me. Once in a while, I would get a tinge of excitement, but it never lasted long.

It was just different this time.

I remember how thrilled I was before Ben was born. Grant's parents had given us the crib that had been Grant's as a baby. Grant had refinished it, and I repainted the little lambs on the headboard. Then I made a brightly flowered quilt for the new baby and a little pillow to match. I wanted everything to be just right.

I'd done the same for Beau and Aber, too. For Beau, I had made a red-and-white gingham with a large teddy bear in the center. And for Aber, one with hobby horses and matching wallpaper in the nursery.

When Ben was born, I spent hours just gazing at his face and getting to know him. And every night I rocked him to sleep. When Beau and Aber arrived, I had more to do but I still made a point of reserving time just for them, time to get to know each of their little personalities. Beau, the sweet little baby who smiled and never seemed to cry. Aber, the raucous little kid whose energy radiated throughout our home from the day he was born.

Time and love are the two essential ingredients of a good relationship between mother and child. I knew I would love this baby. I carried love around inside me. But what about time?

How would I ever find the time to develop that closeness with this new baby? How would I find the energy? I seemed to have been walking around in a permanent state of exhaustion over the last several months. I knew that part of it was due to lack of sleep. But mostly I was emotionally drained from trying to give Ben all my support and good cheer. Every day.

Babies can sense things. I knew that. Wouldn't this new baby know immediately that its mother's heart was all tied up in knots over another child? How could I be there for Ben, pleasant and loving, when I had been up half the night with a new infant?

The dark thoughts, the fears would creep up on me at night in the hospital room like unspoken confessions— thoughts I'd never shared with anyone, thoughts I'd never allowed myself to explore.

We would turn off the television. Ben would say his prayers. And we would telephone Grant to say good night. Then I would kiss Ben, and get into the cot near his bed to go to sleep.

Sometimes I was so exhausted I couldn't fall asleep. Other times I'd crash into oblivion only to wake up in the middle of the night and find myself unable to sleep again. Then, with my eyes wide open in the timeless, eerie yellow light of the nurses' call button, I'd listen to the rhythmic whoosh of Ben's pump, and my darkest thoughts would come out of the shadows to haunt me.

Night after night, the fears would come back. Only the order in which they appeared in my mind would change.

What if this baby were a boy? What if it were another hemophiliac? I had always told everyone I could manage. But it was getting harder as the boys got older and more active.

But it wasn't likely I'd have another boy, was it? Four boys, four straight in a row. Certainly not four hemophiliacs. Besides, this baby inside me was Chelsea. I had told myself that for months now. As if believing it would make it so.

Besides, what could I do about it if it weren't a girl? Nothing. Nothing at all but love my fourth son. I knew I would. It wasn't that I didn't want this child. I did. But I didn't see how I could possibly manage everything. I didn't see how my own physical and emotional stamina would stand up to the long days and nights that I knew lay ahead.

I had been a mother three times over and I knew what those first months were like. I remembered that miraculous but sometimes trying process of tuning two bodies to one cycle. A cycle that meant constant attention and almost no sleep.

And this was just the fourth child.

What about the child after that and the child after that . . . how many more were there? How far were we still from our goal of eight? This was only four. How could I handle twice as many as I had now?

For months these questions had been resounding in my

mind. And the sicker Ben became, the louder the questions became.

As I lay there on the cot next to Ben's bed, I thought about that day Grant and I had walked around the golf course and how we had talked about, dreamed about eight children.

But that was before the hemophilia. And before the AIDS. It wasn't that I didn't want a large family. I did. Or that I didn't have love enough for eight children. I did. But I didn't have the stamina. Not now. Not anymore.

Even then, I had told Grant I could never stand to lose a child. I knew it somehow. And just having Ben sick, having that loss staring me in the face every day, had changed me. I wasn't the same young girl who had been on that golf course. I was a grown woman, still filled with hope, but now I knew heartache all too well.

I had to take control of my life. I, Chris, had to make a decision. I had thought about it for a long time and I had decided that the best thing for me to do would be to have an operation so that I wouldn't get pregnant again.

I had to talk to Grant.

I had to tell him our dream was gone. That AIDS was robbing us not only of our first-born child but of children yet to be conceived.

There was no other way.

And the worst part of it all was that as certain as I was now, in the unsettling night of this hospital room, that this decision was right, I wondered if the time would come, one or three or seven years from now, when I would regret it. Ben would be cured, or be gone. And I would want my dream back. And it would be too late.

But some instinct deep inside me told me this was the right choice. There was no other choice.

Grant and I had our talk one night at Ronald McDonald House when he came up to the hospital to see us. It was very late. I was getting ready for bed and Grant was getting ready to go spend the night on the cot in Ben's room.

"I've been thinking, Grant . . ."

"About what?"

"About our family. What would you think if we didn't have any more children . . . ?"

"But I thought you wanted eight."

"I did. I do. But I don't think we can handle any more. Do you?"

Grant was tired. There were deep circles under his eyes. I could see this wasn't the time to be talking about something so important. But there wasn't any time anymore when we weren't tired. And I could see Grant looking back at me thinking exactly the same thing.

"I've been thinking that we should be thankful for just how much we've been blessed with these boys," I said. "Especially when they get older and are more active and have more bleeds."

"I know this is a hard decision for you," Grant said. "We don't have to have any more children if you don't want to. I'll go along with whatever you decide."

He kissed me good night and went out the door. For ten

years we had been dreaming of having eight children. But now that dream was over.

*　　*　　*

As October wore on, we learned to care for Ben's Hickman. Grant drove up after work when he could to join in. Then he'd drive back to Carmel after midnight.

The hospital staff had suggested we could leave Ben at Stanford until after the baby was born. That would have been easier in some ways. But it meant keeping our family apart. I just felt I couldn't bear having our family divided any longer. I was determined we would all be together at home when the baby was due.

With the help of an organization called Stanford Home Treatment Services and the hospital, it was arranged. We would have a bank of nurses come in to learn how to care for Ben. They would be oriented and taught the details of his regimen and the care of the Hickman. Grant and I would hook him up at night. And then one of these nurses would come in each night around 10:00 P.M. and stay with him all night. At 6:00 A.M. another nurse would relieve her for a couple of hours until I could get Beau and Aber ready for the day. She would draw blood—every day—to take to the hospital for testing, and unhook the pumps. Then I would take over with Ben, tending to his personal needs and changing his Hickman dressing.

It would be complicated. But Ben would be able to live

at home again. And our family would be able to live together. Finally, after six months of constant separations, we would be home.

By the time Ben came home, the hollows in his cheeks had filled in. I could no longer see the skeleton under his skin. It was almost as if time were running backward. Ben had come back. Old Ben. That's what we called him.

And with Ben's weight gain came Ben's spirit, Ben's enthusiasm. Even—ironically, now that Ben didn't need it—Ben's appetite.

The night we got home, he came into the kitchen when I was making chicken wings.

"Ummm, smells like Gramma's," he said. "I'm hungry."

I set a place at the table for five, as I used to, and Ben ate with us. Just as if it were the most natural thing in the world. Just as if it had been the night before that he'd had his last dinner, instead of the month before. He didn't eat much, but he kept it down.

But even though Ben had begun looking a lot like his old self, he had changed inside. He had begun to mature rapidly after his diagnosis. Even the doctors and nurses had commented on it. His manner and his speech seemed like those of someone far older than seven or eight.

He never complained about being hooked up to his Hickman at night. He seemed to take an almost scientific interest in the intricate procedures it required.

Beau was curious about Ben's Hickman and came in to watch the first night I hooked him up.

"Ooh, gross!" he said.

"Well, you don't have to look," Ben said.

Beau walked away, sat on the other bed for a minute, and then came back.

"Does it hurt?" he asked Ben.

"No. It's a little itchy but it makes me feel better."

"Better enough to go out 'n' play like before?"

"Sure. Wanna ride bikes tomorrow?"

"Gee, Ben, really?"

"Sure."

It had been less than a month since Ben had asked me to sell his bike. I hadn't done it yet. I suppose I had been putting it off in the hope that he would be able to ride again after all. But now that he wanted to, I was afraid for him. What if he fell and landed on the Hickman? I bit my tongue and didn't say anything. I couldn't spoil this for Ben—or Beau.

The next morning, the boys took their bikes out of the garage, and we all went outside to watch. Ben pushed off on unsteady legs. But pretty soon he was up and riding, and Beau was right behind him. Grant and Aber and I were all cheering from the front yard.

It was wonderful to see Ben like this again. Cheerful, happy, doing things he could do before. Even though he was still very frail, it was almost as though he were back to normal. I'd never seen anyone go through such a miraculous recovery. It was almost as if the Hickman had given us back our son.

The next Friday night was the Halloween party at church. But when I went to try Ben's costume on that morning,

I was astonished to find he couldn't pull up his black silk pants. Ben had gained nearly fifteen pounds in a month. After all the careful measuring and choosing of fabric, I'd have to remake the pants.

Never before had I enjoyed sewing anything twice.

Ben wrote the longest essay of all the entries in his journal that day. It read:

> Today it is halloween and it is a cheerful day. Well I think it is about time I told you my list for today first I'm going to the Hospital to have blood drawn, than I'm going home again while my mom does my costume. I'm going to watch my cartoons. Then at 6:30 we are going to a Halloween party than at 9:30 we are going home again and then I get hooked up to my machine and then I go to bed. And wake up in the morning again and I hope that I wake up cheerful and Happy.

At the bottom, he drew a jack-o'-lantern, a ghost, and a very realistic bat with a sticker over its face that read "Super Fun Day!"

It was with pride that I dressed my little boys up in their costumes that night. Beau was a robot. And Aber was a knight in shining armor.

Ben, of course, was a Ninja warrior. He put on two T-shirts, so no one would be able to see the outline of his catheter underneath.

Ben was on his own for the first time in perhaps five months that night. At times a funny little robot and a stiff little knight with a spray-painted cardboard sword trailed along beside him. Ben was once again the big brother.

That Halloween was the last time I can remember Aber asking if Ben was all better now.

I knew Ben wasn't all better. I knew it wasn't a recovery. The doctors had warned us the Hickman wasn't a cure for AIDS.

But, on the other hand, why should I overlook the obvious? Ben was better. A lot better. I had seen people who were dying before. And those people were on one-way streets, their bodies deteriorating day by day until finally they died. But Ben had gone to the brink of death and had turned around and walked back again.

So, I began to hope again, began to ask myself another set of questions.

Was it possible that we had weathered the worst of this? Could it be that we were on the verge of being granted the miracle that we all had clung to so fervently? Could this ingenious little device keep Ben alive indefinitely, or at least long enough for the researchers to find a cure?

Was it possible that Ben wasn't going to die after all?

I kept trying to remind myself that time with Ben was what was important. I had to tell myself: Accept this time with Ben and enjoy him while you can. But don't think you can keep him, because you can't.

We were supposed to have nursing from 10:00 P.M. until 10:00 A.M. the next day. But sometimes they couldn't find anyone to come in. Grant would help sometimes. But he wasn't as knowledgeable about the procedures as I was, and he was already working long hours just to pay the mortgage.

So it would fall to me to adjust the flow of the nutrition into Ben's body, to help him to the bathroom, to change the sheets when accidents happened.

I remember sitting there one day in a daze of exhaustion. The baby was due in less than two weeks. If I was tired now, how would I ever be able to cope with a newborn waking every few hours of the night and day?

This should have been a happy time, a joyful time. But AIDS had come along and robbed us of the joy.

About ten days before my due date, Grant drove me to my obstetrician's appointment. He had always come to my appointments with me when he could, but this time he had been able to come to only a couple of them. As we were driving, I asked him to pull over to the side of the road.

"Please," I said.

I could feel tears and anger welling up inside me as he stopped.

"Oh, Grant, nothing has turned out the way it was supposed to. Nothing. Look what's happening to us. Is this the way we thought it would be? What's happened to all our plans?"

"Oh, Chris, don't feel so bad. Look, we're on the way to the doctor's office and we're about to have a wonderful new baby, and. . . ."

He turned off the engine and waited for me to say something.

"All I ever wanted was a happy family. That's all. Was that too much to ask? I mean that one thing was all I ever wanted. Now, everything is so complicated. When I was little, I just wanted my parents to stay together. And they didn't. They got a divorce. I just wanted a sister so I would have someone to talk to. Someone like me. But I got three brothers. . . ."

I could see the concern on Grant's face. He was going to try to comfort me, and I didn't want to be comforted. I just wanted to cry and get this out. Once and for all. And I wanted him to go through it with me.

"And then I got married and we were going to have eight children. And then I wanted a girl. Two girls, at least, so they could be sisters. But I got three boys. And we sure didn't count on them being hemophiliacs, did we? And we sure didn't count on one of them getting AIDS, did we, Grant?"

"Oh, Chris, I know how hard this is on you," he said, moving to put his arm around me over the big space between the two front seats in the van.

"No, I don't think you do!"

I didn't mean to hurt him. But I hurt so much myself.

"I always knew the one thing I could never handle in my whole life was for one of my children to die. And Ben is going to die. It's not fair. And we're going to have another baby. And what am I supposed to feel? Excitement? The only thing I know for sure is I can't have any more children. I just couldn't handle any more."

"I know what you're saying, Chris. It's fine with me."

"You said you'd 'go along' with anything I wanted. But that's not enough. You've got to go through this decision with me."

"I will go through it with you, Chris. The only thing I want to know is if you're really sure."

"No, I'm not sure!"

I needed Grant to realize how much this mattered to me, how hard a decision this was for me.

"Come on, Chris. Don't worry. Our boys are terrific. It's not that big a deal if we don't have any more children."

"Not that big a deal? If it's not that big a deal, why don't you have the operation?"

He got defensive.

"Well, sure. Why not?"

I wasn't trying to get Grant to have the operation. I didn't care who had it. I just wanted him to understand that this was the hardest decision of my whole life, that one quick little conversation before bedtime wasn't enough when it came to giving up a dream you had dreamed your whole life. It hurt me so much inside to make that decision that I think I needed Grant to hurt too so he'd know what I was going through.

And I had hurt him. I could see it in his eyes. He was puzzled. Why was I attacking him when he hadn't done anything except agree with me?

I couldn't say I was sorry because I wasn't. But I could show him I loved him, because I did. More than anything in the world. I leaned over and put my arms around him and cried on his chest, and he comforted me. He was the only thing that had turned out right, more right than I had ever imagined.

When I gave the doctor the signed form that night, authorizing the tubal ligation, he asked me if I was really sure I wanted to do it. And I answered, "Yes. I'm sure."

And I was.

That decision meant much more to me than the fact that we would have only half the children we wanted. It was a reckoning. A recognition that in order to gain something, you often have to give something up.

What I had given up, I realize now, was nothing less than a part of myself. That part of me that was young and carefree and thought I could do anything. I would never be that Chris again. I would never again dream so carelessly. I would never again assume I could do what I had never tried. I would, from now on, be aware of dangers around me, bad things that even goodwill could not conquer.

But for all that loss of innocence, I had gained something too. I took back control of my life. I had lost the control, let myself be blown back and forth from day to day by the particular state of Ben's health. I knew there would be even harder times ahead. But I had steeled myself to handle them.

When I called my mother the next day to ask her to come up for that visit she'd suggested when we were moving, it wasn't a child asking a mother for help. It was a grown daughter inviting a grandmother to share in the joy of getting ready for the arrival of a new baby.

I was ready, now, to be excited about the baby. And there was nobody like my mom for getting me in the mood. Grant had gotten the crib down from the attic and was searching for the box of baby clothes when she arrived.

"Forget the old clothes," she said. "What this baby needs is some new things. Get a baby-sitter, Chris. We're going shopping."

It was like old times, that day. Like the times before Ben was born, when Mom was so thrilled about the prospect of her first grandchild. She took me to lunch at a little restaurant I liked and then to a special baby store that was more expensive than Grant and I could really afford. Since I hadn't had time to make a quilt, the first thing we picked out was a beautiful new blanket.

❊   ❊   ❊

Less than a week later, I went into labor. I called Mom and Ralph, and they promised to be up later that evening to take care of Beau and Aber. Then I called the nursing service. I had let them know in advance that we'd need three days of round-the-clock nursing as soon as the labor began.

But, by late afternoon, the nurse still hadn't come. Grant called the nursing service, only to be told again that a nurse was on her way. It wasn't until 7:00 P.M. that she finally arrived.

When she walked in the door, I could feel a knot tighten in my stomach. It was somebody we didn't even know. Not our usual nurses. Not Heather or Nancy. A woman who had had to come to the initial session at our home with other nurses to learn about the Hickman. But she had never cared for Ben. Not once. She was a stranger to him.

I hooked Ben up for the night, giving her careful instructions between contractions—"contraptions," Ben called them—and imploring her to follow carefully the detailed chart I had taped to the closet door.

I tucked Ben in and kissed him good-night.

"Good luck, Mom," he said. "I hope it's a boy."

Nothing about this labor was like those before it. With each previous birth, Grant and I had studied Lamaze techniques. We had practiced together the breathing patterns that would help me through the worst of the contractions. Each of those labors had gone well. I had felt confident and clearheaded, despite the pain. I hadn't needed any drugs with any of the births.

From the beginning, the contractions seemed much harder than any of those I had felt in my previous births. I couldn't remember any of the breathing techniques. And the contractions kept sneaking up on me. It just felt all wrong. I felt nervous and unsettled. I couldn't concentrate. I kept thinking about Ben instead of the baby.

"Grant . . . I can't think . . . What if the nurse doesn't set the rate of flow right?" I asked him between contractions. "They said Ben could . . . could have a heart attack if it's wrong."

"She'll do fine. Don't worry. Just pretend there is nothing else in this world right now but you and me and this baby.

Just us. Just concentrate on our baby. We're going to have a baby. Think about that. A new baby."

He offered me some ice chips.

"I can't concentrate, Grant. I don't remember how to do it."

I could feel the next contraction coming on.

Grant took hold of my hands firmly.

"Look at me, honey. You can do this. You've done it before and you'll do it again. And if it gets too hard, we'll get you some medicine. So don't worry. Just concentrate. Breathe with me. Look at me. Like this . . . That's right. Breathe! In and out. Breathe!"

I watched his face and I breathed as he breathed, grateful for the moment not to have to think.

If it hadn't been for Grant, I never would have made it through those prior births without medication. And I could feel his strength now. He was the most wonderful, loving husband I could imagine. Someone who always came through for me when I really needed him to. Always.

"I, I love you, Grant," I told him when I could speak again.

"I know."

The labor went on and the pain got worse. I couldn't think of anything anymore. Not the baby. Not Ben. Not Grant coaching me to breathe right. I had always had a high tolerance for pain, something I suppose you're born with or you're not. But now I couldn't take it anymore. I was physically and emotionally used up.

I gave up, and asked for medication.

And even when I got it, the pain didn't go away.

Finally, about 3:00 A.M., I could feel the urge to push the baby out. The exhilaration of birth was upon me now, I could feel it. The baby was on its way.

And I wanted it. I wanted the baby. I couldn't wait to see my baby. Grant and the doctor and the nurses were cheering me on. The baby was coming.

I could feel its head come out of me.

"Chris, it's got a whole lot of hair," Grant said. "I think we got our wish. It's a girl!"

I felt the rest of the baby come out, and the doctor turned her over.

"No, wait," the doctor said. "It's a boy! A handsome little baby boy."

Finally, I let go of my tears and forgot the pain. I was crying, I was so happy. I didn't care if it was a girl or a boy. Was it a girl I had wanted really? Or was it this wonderful new little boy? I just wanted my baby. And having that baby was every bit as wonderful as having Ben and Beau and Aber had been.

I still had all that love inside me, after all. It had just been locked up somewhere, out of reach.

* * *

We named our fourth son Daniel Kimball Oyler. He weighed eight pounds, four ounces. His birthday was November 6, 1985.

Dr. Penn stopped by to see us and check out his newest little Oyler patient that afternoon.

He was beaming as he walked into the room.

"I just got the test results," he said. "The baby is healthy in every way. A perfectly healthy, normal little boy—no hemophilia."

I felt a rush of relief wash through me. Grant was beaming as he held the little baby in his arms.

Ben had gotten his little brother.

And we had gotten our first miracle.

6

"I Want to Go Home"

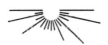

THE MOMENT we brought Danny home from the hospital, it was as if someone had opened a big window and let fresh air in. Fresh air that seemed to blow away all the anxieties of the long months that had preceded his birth.

As soon as we walked in the front door, the boys all rushed to see him. They could barely contain their excitement as, one by one, they peeked inside the fresh white blanket trimmed in blue. Yes, blue. It was the blanket my mother and I had bought the day she took me shopping for the baby. And as much as I had thought about and planned for a little girl, I had bought a white blanket with blue trim.

I hadn't even thought about the color. I just bought blue as if all Oyler babies were boys.

And Ben had the baby brother he wanted.

"Can I hold him, Mom? Can I?" Ben asked.

"Of course, you can. Sit down on the sofa."

Ben sat down. Beau and Aber plopped down right beside him to make sure they got their turns.

I unfolded the blanket and placed Danny in Ben's arms. Ben smiled with pride as Danny wrapped his little fingers around Ben's thumb.

"He's so little," Ben said, almost whispering. "Look at his tiny fingers."

I just stood and stared at them. Danny's bright little round eyes reminded me so much of Ben's when he was a baby.

Here was this miraculously alive little being. What a gift he was. To me. To the whole family. But especially to Ben. Of all the things on Ben's list of "things to look forward to" that we had made up so many months before, this was the one that mattered. Really mattered.

"And he'll really never have to get a shot?" Beau asked.

"Not factor," I answered. "He'll have to get other kinds of shots. But he'll never have to have Factor VIII shots."

Beau marveled at the very idea.

"My turn to hold him," Aber said.

"I'm not done yet," Ben said.

"You have to share," Aber negotiated.

With three little boys vying for toys, *share* was a word I had used often. And even as a preschooler, Aber had quickly learned that fairness was a good argument.

Danny meant something special to Aber, meant he would never have to be the baby again.

But long after the newness of having a baby around wore off for Beau and Aber, Ben still loved to hold Danny. They seemed to have their own special connection, those two.

Danny brought such joy to my life. Joy that somehow erased the sorrow I hadn't been able to fight off on my own.

Our bonding was immediate and complete. When I held him in my arms, I was a new mother again. He needed me and I needed him and our dependence on each other was life-giving. He brought forth a surge of warm, unrestrained love in me that I had almost forgotten.

His perfect health was my assurance that he would live, that he would grow up healthy and strong.

He was my promise that the future would come and that it would be good.

Those first few weeks were sheer bliss. After my stay in the hospital, I felt rested for the first time in months. Grant took time off from work. He cooked and took care of the boys while I took care of Danny.

And Ben was feeling good.

There were days when he'd wake feeling almost like his old self. "I can do it, Mom," he'd say with a note of impatience if I tried to help him dress.

There were so many things that we had checked off as things that Ben would never be able to do again that suddenly, because of the Hickman, he felt like doing. Like going to the park and playing on the gym equipment. We hadn't been there since the day I had told Ben about Jessica. Now he wanted to go.

When we got home, he wrote in his journal: "I went on everything—twice."

Ben volunteered to do odd jobs around the house so he could earn money to go to Oscar Hossenfellder's. He even helped Grant lay a wood floor. And when Aber said that what he wanted to do for his fourth birthday was play miniature golf, Ben couldn't wait.

Things started to feel normal again. And I was so encouraged.

Ironically, I found it more difficult to answer Ben's questions about his illness when he was feeling good than I did when he was sick.

"When am I going to get better?" Ben asked one night when I was hooking him up to the machine.

"We don't know, Ben. I wish we did. You know AIDS is pretty serious and the doctors are trying as hard as they can to help you. But we're going to have to wait and see if they can come up with some new medicine that will help." *And we need to pray extra hard for you to get better,* I thought.

"Mom, does Heavenly Father want me to get better?" Ben asked.

What was I supposed to tell Ben? I myself didn't know what God's will was. I couldn't say to Ben, straight out, that I didn't know if he was going to live or die. Ben knew that people were dying from AIDS. My job was to get him through every day with a little bit of hope.

"Heavenly Father loves you very much, Benny, and I'm sure He wants you to feel better. But sometimes we can't always tell what is in His mind. Sometimes we just have to wait and trust Him that it will be all right."

Ben's relatively good state of health was puzzling to Beau and Aber too. They never knew quite how to treat him from one day to the next. One day Beau came running in from outside to watch "GI Joe" on television and found Ben in the living room watching "Transformers."

"It's my turn," Beau announced.

"I was here first," Ben said.

"Well, you've been sitting here all day," Beau responded. "Give somebody else a chance."

"I've been waiting all day for 'Transformers.' You can go outside and play with your friends. I can't."

That stopped Beau cold. If Ben was sick, he didn't want to hurt him. He knew special rules somehow applied. But Ben looked a lot better to him now. So Beau didn't know what he should do.

"Mom!" Beau called for help.

I came out of the kitchen to settle the argument, ruling that it was Beau's turn. One of my daily struggles throughout Ben's sickness was trying to meet Ben's needs without favoring him over the other boys too much. It hurt me so to see them argue when I knew how precious their time together was. How precious and how limited.

"When your Uncle Randy and I were little, we used to fight all the time," I told them. "And then all of a sudden we grew up and didn't see each other. And we missed each other. So it's important that you show people how much you love them whenever you have a chance."

I felt so sorry for Ben sometimes. He was not only sick, he was bored. He missed school. And sports. And break dancing. And so many things he had loved.

The tutor won Ben over the day she arrived at our house, carrying a bag full of what Ben called "wooden knots." They were bulbs. Daffodil and tulip bulbs. And Ben was fascinated.

He had never seen bulbs before and he couldn't believe that something beautiful could actually grow from these ugly little knots.

I watched the two of them planting the bulbs in the backyard. Ben was having such a good time. But I wondered why she had chosen bulbs. Bulbs took so long to bloom. Wouldn't it have been easier just to plant seeds or small plants? As much as I hated the thought, I worried that Ben might not live long enough to see them bloom.

Every day he went out to check on them. Waiting to see the first sprig of green. With those bulbs, the tutor had given Ben something truly special. A renewed interest in life and growing.

But no adult, no brother, no parent could make up for the fact that Ben really didn't have any friends his own age to play with. Some younger neighbor boys would come over to visit sometimes, but if Ben started coughing or throwing up, they'd run off and leave Ben stranded.

We ran into some of Ben's old friends one day at the soccer field when Beau had a game.

"Why don't you go over and say hi?" I suggested to Ben.

"I don't want to," Ben said. "Besides, they won't remember me."

"Just say 'Hi, I'm Ben Oyler, remember me?'"

It took a little encouragement, but finally he did. The boys were classmates of his from his old school, but they didn't recognize him.

"You're Ben Oyler?" one boy asked, in disbelief.

"Yeah, I am," Ben said. "I've just been sick. That's all. Remember that boy at River School with AIDS? That's me."

One of the boys backed up immediately and I could see the hurt look on Ben's face. I got up quickly with Danny and walked over.

I asked the boys if they knew what AIDS was. And the one who backed away said he knew you could catch it. Easy. And you could die from it too. So I talked to them about it for a few minutes and explained that there were only a few ways to get AIDS—none of which were by playing. It wasn't something you catch like a cold. Even his brothers and his parents couldn't get it being around him all the time.

There are moments in life that happen almost as if by magic and this was one of them. I watched as the little boy who had been the most scared did something for Ben that I, despite all my love for him, would never have thought to do. He gave him a piece of paper, and showed him how to make a throwing star.

Ben's eyes lit up. He instantly became engrossed in the folded paper. Ben had helped me make dozens of Valentines, patiently cutting out paper doilies I pasted onto red construction paper. But this was different. This was play. And it was healing to Ben's soul. I could see it. I slipped away when I heard Ben talking Ninja warriors with the boys.

"I've got a real throwing star at home!"

For a whole hour, Ben and the boys made throwing stars. Ben wrote down one of the boys' phone numbers, but I knew, once they got home, their parents' will would prevail. And that they probably would never be allowed to play with the little boy with AIDS again.

Seeing Ben with the other boys did my heart good but seeing him next to healthy boys his own age was hard on me. The other boys were a head taller than he was now. Ben had stopped growing. Next to them, he still looked like a seven-year-old. A seven-year-old with a puffy little face. Ben had put on weight, but the weight looked unnatural.

It's no wonder they didn't recognize him. He wasn't the Ben Oyler they remembered. Not the Old Ben.

As autumn wore on, Ben's health began to deteriorate, little by little. His cough grew deeper. And his stomach cramps came back.

He also seemed to be staggering a little, and I began to fear AIDS was attacking his brain. Was nothing off limits to this awful disease? We took Ben up to the hospital for a day of brain scans. But the doctors couldn't find anything wrong. With AIDS, they said, things happen "for no apparent reason."

Our bills mounted, and Grant had to keep up his work schedule. The exhaustion that had been so familiar to me before Danny was born began to set in again.

Sometimes, when Ben's illness became too depressing or the demands of the day too trying to face, I would go into my room and close the door. I'd sit in my rocking chair with Danny and rock him just because I needed the warmth of his little body next to mine.

I wanted to shut out the world and just be a mother to this little baby. For the first time, I could feel myself withdrawing from our family circle—just for a few precious moments. Not because I didn't love my husband or my children just as much as I always had. But because I didn't want to face what I had to face.

My mind kept coming back to Jessica, and how she had gone into a coma before dying. Could that happen to Ben? Could he slip away without our ever having the chance to sit down with him and really prepare him for the life we believed awaited him beyond this one? Could time run out on us even as we were trying to keep hope alive for Ben?

Grant and I decided to call all the boys together one night for a family home evening. We rolled Ben's portable pumps into the living room. We began with a favorite song and then a prayer. I held Danny in my arms, and Beau and Aber settled down slowly as Grant began the lesson.

"You know how thankful we are for Danny and how glad we are that he joined our family," he said.

"Yeah!" all three of them said in unison.

"Well, let's talk about what it was like when Danny was born," Grant continued. The boys didn't take their eyes off Grant.

"You see, before Danny was born, he was a spirit . . . sort of like your hand." Grant raised his hand and wriggled his fingers. "And when he was born . . ." Grant pulled a glove out of his pocket and slipped it on his hand. "When he was born, his spirit got a body . . . like this glove."

He wriggled his fingers again inside the glove. "It was his

spirit that gave his body life just like my hand gives this glove life. Do you understand?"

The boys were all fascinated. None of them made a sound. Grant paused and studied each of their faces to make sure they truly did understand.

"And when you die," he continued, "it's as if the body just slips off again." He removed the glove from his hand and placed it on the table in front of the boys. They stared at the lifeless object.

"But the spirit continues," he said, wriggling the fingers on his hand once again. "You see, our bodies may die, but our spirits never die. Our spirits will live forever."

"But I don't wanna die," Beau said.

"Nobody really wants to die," Grant said. "We like it here. That's good. This world is a great place. But dying is nothing to be afraid of either. We're all born and sooner or later, we all die."

"It's just the cycle of life, Beau," I said. "Every living thing is born and every living thing dies. Every person. Every animal. Every plant. It's all part of God's plan. You don't have to be afraid of it, Beau, because dying is really just another part of living. After you die, you just go on to a different kind of life in heaven."

Ben was quiet. I remember wondering what he was thinking, wondering if he knew the lesson was for him.

❀   ❀   ❀

Christmas was just a few weeks away. It had always been my favorite time of year. A time to love, a time to reach out to others.

I sat down one morning with Ben to write out a list—this time of things that we could do for other people. Gifts to make and deliver, people to visit. Homemade ice cream for Dr. Penn. A wreath for the Rasbands' door. And a few presents we would make and leave as a surprise and nobody would know. But I didn't know if he would be up to it all. I didn't even know if I would be up to it. And I didn't see now how I would find the time.

I had always felt that a mother sets the whole tone of Christmas for a family. But what sort of mood would I set this year? How could I be cheerful and warm when I could see Ben's suffering coming back? I wasn't even sure if we'd be home or back in the hospital for Christmas.

We did put out the little winter scene that had sat on our family piano every Christmas since I was small. And added a little electric train to go around the miniature city with little cardboard houses I remembered from my childhood. I baked cookies. I made ornaments and a wreath. Ben helped me deliver our little presents.

For the first time since we had been married, Grant and I had the large picture window I had always wanted for a Christmas tree. That was one of the things that had made me fall in love with the house. But now, even with a big tree twinkling in the window at night, I longed for Christmases of the past with a little tree jammed into the corner of our duplex.

One of Ben's favorite home nurses, Heather, took Ben on a date to Oscar Hossenfellder's to share a hot fudge sundae and a merry-go-round ride. But what thrilled Ben the most was her present: a pair of break-dancing gloves. He wore them every day.

I began to feel as though we were on a roller-coaster ride. We had been riding high after the Hickman and now we were plunging downward again. I just hoped Ben could hang on.

The night before Christmas Eve, he walked straight into a doorjamb and fell on the floor, almost knocking himself out. I made a call to the hospital, but I knew there wasn't anything else they could tell me. They had done all the tests. They could find no cause for his neurological problems.

That night, I sat down with a heavy heart and wrote in my journal, "I am frightened that Ben may die soon. I pray every day for a cure for AIDS." When I asked Ben what he wanted for Christmas, his response came as a complete surprise. Violin lessons! He'd never even mentioned a violin before. And I didn't think he had the strength to hold a violin, much less to learn to play one. But if he wanted violin lessons, I was going to do everything in my power to get them for him.

One day before Christmas we went shopping for a violin and found a small, old one at an antique shop on Cannery Row. Then I set out to find a teacher so he could start right after the holidays. The first one turned me down flat, said she'd have to check with her doctor first. If she really thought she could get AIDS from teaching the violin, she wasn't the teacher for Ben.

After a series of phone calls, I found the perfect teacher, an older woman who loved the instrument and would be both suitably understanding and suitably strict. It was important to Ben and me that she treat him as normally as possible. So, the violin lessons became the next thing to look forward to.

We didn't buy many toys that Christmas. They didn't seem to matter somehow. On Christmas Eve, we read from the Bible about the Christ Child's birth. And we sang Christmas carols on Christmas Eve. But they didn't resonate in my heart the way they always had before.

We opened presents as usual on Christmas morning. But while Beau and Aber were wildly thrashing through paper and boxes, Ben sat quietly, watching his brothers.

Finally, Ben stood up and walked over to each of us, giving us a little hand-wrapped package and he watched as we opened them up. Inside were little ceramic figurines he had made in scouts. A bear for Beau, a dog for Aber, a red heart that said "I love you, Mom" for me. And for Grant a special gift, a clay statue Ben had made at the hospital, a remarkable likeness of Abraham Lincoln, beard and stovepipe hat and all, reading a book.

But those little gifts, made with incredible detail and love, meant the world to us. They still do. I suppose we appreciated it all the more because of the love and energy that Ben had put into them.

As I looked around the messy living room that morning,

I thought about how lucky I was to be a mother. Each of the boys was special, each was different. Ben, the creative little boy with stamina beyond his years. Beau, the deep quiet one with the twinkling blue eyes. And Aber, who had somehow during this last year—almost when I wasn't looking—stopped being a toddler.

And Danny—Danny had renewed my faith in life itself. I think he was God's way of telling me Yes, you can do this, you can be a mother. To Danny, to Aber, to Beau. And yes, to Ben too. I could almost hear a little voice in the back of my mind comforting me, saying: Why do you suppose I gave you Ben?

And then I remembered the Holy Ghost. I had almost forgotten that He wasn't only for children.

Ben learned to play one song, "Hot Cross Buns," on his violin before we had to take him back up to the hospital. The Hickman had given him four whole months at home. But now the medication we were giving him at home was no longer enough to take away his pain.

Ben had suffered from almost constant vomiting, and constant diarrhea, for more than seven months. And now he was in agonizing pain, doubling over from cramps.

This time the doctors diagnosed pancreatitis, an extraordinarily painful disease. They increased his pain medication and inserted a tube through his nose and down his throat to his stomach to remove some of the gastric juices that were causing part of the pain.

Ben still had some good days, but there were far more bad

days now than before. And he was very, very ill on those days. He had been so well so recently that the change was doubly hard on him. He would get excited about looking at a new airplane model. Then his hands would shake so much that he couldn't finish putting it together. He wrote in his journal only once during February and March: "Today I'm in the hospital." That was all. His writing was so feeble it was hard to read.

Days passed, and weeks.

Sometimes I would think, *This can't go on. There must be an end somewhere to Ben's suffering.* And then I would remind myself that time was our ally in this battle for Ben's life, that every new day meant more research was being done on AIDS.

I could feel myself growing numb.

The world didn't seem real anymore. Our family never seemed to be in one place together anymore. Grant and I hardly ever saw each other. He was working. I was at the hospital. Beau and Aber were usually with friends or relatives, and I found myself having fantasy fears every now and then that they too had gotten sick, even though I knew better. I yearned to see their healthy faces and hear their happy voices.

I wrote in my journal one night that Danny was the only thing that was keeping me sane.

Grant and I had to bring our family back together again. But how? If only we knew how long Ben would be sick . . . If only we knew Ben was going to be at the hospital like this for another year, or more, we could move to Palo Alto. Enroll Beau in school nearby. Open up a new business for Grant here.

That was what we wanted to do. To plan our lives as if our hopes would one day be realized and Ben would get well. Somehow I had had it in the back of my mind that the Hickman would give Ben three more years. I don't know why. I just did. If that were the case, we would have to rearrange our lives around this hospital.

But what if Ben were to die sooner? What if Ben were to die, as the statistics told us he might, before May?

I couldn't think about that. I couldn't because I had to hope that Ben would live. And yet, as awful as it sounded, Grant and I had to make practical decisions about our family life that took into account the very real possibility that Ben would die.

It was an awful contradiction: to hope for life, yet to prepare for death.

Finally, we decided to take Beau out of school, and bring him and Aber up to the hospital to stay with me. Grant would work Tuesdays, Wednesdays, and Thursdays and come up for four-day weekends with us at the hospital. The hours he worked those three days were unbelievably long.

One night, he got home about midnight after spending a week with us at the hospital and was trying to sleep when he heard noises in the kitchen. He got up and opened a cupboard door and found river rats running around inside. It had rained all weekend and the river by our house had risen. The rats had invaded.

Then, all alone in our little house, he told me, he got out his BB gun and opened the cupboard doors, and crouched down behind the kitchen counter and shot at them as if in an arcade.

"I'm sorry, Chris," he told me. "I don't know what came over me. But I stopped when they got to the shelf with your good china in it."

"I'm glad you drew the line somewhere," I joked with him. This didn't sound like the sensible Grant I knew, taking BB-gun potshots at rats at 1:00 A.M.

The stress was beginning to show. Anger and sadness and the frightening inability to make Ben any better were getting to all of us.

Even Beau.

The school psychologist had talked to Beau a few times. And he recommended that Beau continue to see a psychologist at the hospital. "It's just helpful to have someone outside the family to talk to," he told me. "Don't worry. You're doing everything right. Just be ready to talk to him whenever he really wants to talk."

That was reassuring. But when did I have time to sit down with Beau, and really talk to him alone? I knew that Beau needed me. I hadn't taken enough time with him, but time was what I had the least of. Ben's illness, Danny's needs, and Aber's propensity for getting into trouble used up all the hours in the day.

When we finally moved up to the hospital, both Beau and Aber were excited. I checked out a big corner room at the Ronald McDonald house, and rolled in some extra beds. You couldn't walk across the room because it was wall-to-wall beds. But to the litte boys, it was like camping out.

Having them with me made me feel better. Finally, we were more like a family. But it was hectic trying to nurse Danny through the night without waking Beau and Aber and trying to find time to sleep myself.

One rainy night about 3:00 A.M. the phone rang. It was a nurse. Ben had vomited up the tube that led to his stomach. Again. They had been putting in successively larger tubes in hopes that the bigger ones would finally stay down. The insertion of those tubes was more painful to Ben than anything else he had ever had done to him. And now they were going to insert a large, adult-size tube.

"He asked if you could come over," the nurse said. "He won't let us put it in without you."

I needed to be with Ben. But I couldn't leave the other boys. Danny had gotten his first immunization the day before and was feverish and fidgety. Beau was asleep. Aber had gone home with Grant.

I didn't know what to do. I felt pulled in so many directions at once. I had thought if I could just get my family in one place, things would be manageable. But here I was, just a few hundred yards from Ben, and I still felt divided. Everybody needed me at once.

"Could you put Ben on the phone?" I asked.

"Mom, it'll hurt," Ben cried. "I don't want them to do it."

"I know it hurts, honey. But Ben, listen to me, I can't leave Danny. He has a temperature and Beau is asleep. I just can't leave them here alone. But if you'll keep the phone right next to your ear I'll stay with you on the phone and talk to you while they're putting the tube in. I'll be right here with you, okay?"

I said a little prayer in Ben's ear: "Please, Heavenly Father, help Ben to be brave."

I nursed Danny to keep him quiet while I talked to Ben on the phone. As I sat there in the dark, I could hear the sounds of my son gagging and coughing as the nurses tried to get the tube down his throat.

"It's okay, Benny. Try to relax. Keep swallowing. I love you, honey. You can do it. I know it must hurt, but you're being so brave . . . you're going to be fine . . . they have to get this tube in to make you feel better . . . it'll all be over in a couple of minutes."

When at last the gagging stopped, I could hear Ben trying to say good-night.

How much more of this could Ben possibly take? It was so unfair for one little boy to suffer so much when he hadn't done anything at all to deserve it. How much more suffering could he bear?

As I hung up the phone, I saw that Danny's hair was soaking wet from my tears. And something stirred under the covers next to me. Beau. Could it be that Beau had heard all this? That Beau was awake?

"Beau?" I whispered.

He didn't say a word.

Everywhere I looked there were things that needed doing.

Not loads of laundry and dishes. But children's emotions that needed shoring up. And here I was, crying in the dark. Pouring energy down the drain in tears.

❊ ❊ ❊

It was Saturday morning. Grant was with Ben. I was downstairs taking a walk with Beau and Aber and Danny when I heard the loudspeaker announce "Stat Room 205!" Room 205. That was Ben's room. I didn't know what the announcement meant, but the tone was urgent. I ran to the closest telephone and frantically called Ben's room. There was no answer. I started running back with the boys when another announcement called for a respiratory unit to Ben's room.

A nurse came down the hall to meet me. She took the boys and told me to hurry to Ben.

I ran down to the room and looked in, and through a throng of doctors and nurses I could see Ben's little body jerking up and down on the bed, over and over and over again. Never, ever, had I seen a body go through such a violent movement.

I just stood there, terrified, while a dozen or more doctors and nurses all worked on Ben at once, trying to give him oxygen and some sort of medicine. My eyes met with Grant's. He was standing next to Ben's bed, holding on to Ben. He motioned for me to come. I pushed my way through the doctors. I had to reach Ben.

Then, abruptly, the seizure stopped and his body went limp on the bed, flat and spent.

Ben, oh Ben. Are you alive?

I took his hand in mine and spoke quietly but deeply, urgently, into his ear. If he was alive, I had to get through to him.

"I love you, Ben, I love you," I said.

I looked up and saw Grant holding Ben's hand on the other side of the bed. His face was as white as a sheet.

"We're here, Ben. Daddy and me. We love you."

"Mom . . . I want to go home."

His voice was barely a whisper.

A nurse looked at me as if to say going home was, of course, out of the question.

"Everything's going to be okay. We love you, Ben," I said.

"Mom, I want to go home."

Ben had to say it twice before I realized what he was saying. He didn't mean Carmel. He meant really going home. We had told Ben dying was like going home. And now he was ready.

"It's okay, honey. I understand. I do."

"Will you come visit me there?"

"Yes, Ben. I will. Someday."

7

"You Won, Ben! You Won!"

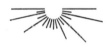

BEN LAY ON THE BED. Lifeless. Eyes closed. A machine measured his breathing. A nurse was assigned to stay with him around the clock. His toys were haphazardly piled in a corner, frantically put there to make room for the emergency equipment.

It was Dr. Glader's day off, but he came in anyway to examine Ben. He explained to us that Ben had had something called a grand mal seizure and was lucky to be alive.

His voice was uncharacteristically heavy. The seizure, he said, was probably brought on because AIDS had attacked Ben's central nervous system. There could be brain damage. Paralysis. Or there could be no aftereffects at all.

He added an antiseizure medicine to Ben's growing list of drugs and told us Ben would probably sleep for a long time. It was the body's way of repairing from the trauma of the seizure. And, he warned, seizures can strike twice.

A vial of emergency medicine, which would help revive him in case of another seizure, was taped to Ben's wall. Just in case.

After we talked to the doctor, Grant and I went back to the lounge to talk to Beau and Aber, to try to explain, as best we could, about Ben.

Aber was watching television. Beau was facing the screen,

looking white as a sheet. He just looked up at us, this little six-year-old, and it was clear he was afraid what we were going to say. And I was so shaken myself it was hard to find my mother's voice, the voice that would tell Beau the truth without scaring him.

"He's asleep right now, Beau," I said.

"What happened to him, Mom?"

Beau came over and I sat him on my lap. And Grant went over to Aber. He was still pretty little. Too little.

"He had something called a seizure, Beau."

"Is that bad?"

"Yes, pretty bad. But it's over now."

Beau just sat there a moment, looking down at his hands, chubby, little first-grader hands.

"Mom, is Ben gonna die?"

Oh, Beau . . . what do I tell you? I could feel a knot rising in my throat. There were so many emotions welling up inside me. I didn't know what to say, didn't even know what I was supposed to say. It was all I could do to try to control my voice so my emotions wouldn't all just spill out in tears. I couldn't let that happen. I couldn't. Beau needed reassurance, desperately needed it.

I had to find the words . . .

I held him closer for a minute and took a deep breath, and said, "I don't know, Beau. We're not sure. I know how hard this is for you. But I don't want you to worry right now, because he's sleeping. He's all right for the moment. He's just very, very tired and he needs to sleep for a while."

"You Won, Ben! You Won!"

"I love Ben, Mommy."

"I know, Beau. I know . . . Beau, I need to get back to Ben. Can you be brave for me now, just for a few more days? And then we'll talk about it some more, okay, honey?"

His little face nodded against my chest.

"I love you, Beau."

I could see the need inside Beau. It was achingly clear. He had been uprooted from everything he knew, his home, his school, and all too often, from his parents.

How long had he been living with that question inside him? How long had he been wondering if his big brother was going to die?

My blouse was wet from his tears. He was my son too. And I loved him very much. But there would be time later. Time to spend with Beau. Time to try heal the pain he was going through now. *Someday I'll make it up to you, Beau. I will. I promise.*

I understood Beau's fear a lot more clearly later. Months later, when he admitted to me that he had sneaked away from the nurses and peeked into Ben's room. He had seen it. The aftermath of the seizure: the throng of doctors, the oxygen machine, nurses forcing the oxygen mask over Ben's face. And, finally, Ben just lying still on the bed.

But that day I didn't have time to sit down and talk to Beau, didn't have time to really sort things out, no matter how much I needed to.

Instead, I had to kiss Beau and Aber good-bye once again,

and watch them go off with some close friends who had happened to come by the hospital for a visit.

For the rest of the day, I sat on one side of Ben's bed and Grant sat on the other. And, together with the duty nurse, we waited. Waited for Ben to wake up. For Ben to have another seizure. For something to happen.

It turned dark, and we had another cot brought in so both of us could stay in Ben's room. But I think Ben was the only one who slept.

Ben was ready to let go; he had told me so himself. His words echoed through my mind: I want to go home. I want to go home.

That was the closest Ben had ever come to talking about his own death. We had developed an understanding, the two of us, that we would keep waging this war without ever talking about how it would end. An unspoken understanding that was covered by the very thinnest veneer of hope. Ben must have been very close to the end to say those words to me.

But what were we supposed to do now? Grant and I were Ben's advocates in this life. What did he want us to do? Just let go? Just an hour before his seizure, Ben had been happily playing with Beau and Aber. The day before, he had been outside in the courtyard finishing up one airplane model and talking about the next model he wanted to buy at Toys-R-Us.

That didn't sound like a boy who was dying, did it? No, that was a boy who was holding on to life.

But now there was the possibility that Ben might die

suddenly. Tonight. Tomorrow. And there was the possibility that he might slip away into a coma like his friend Jessica, technically alive but not really living. Half alive. Half Ben. That, I knew, neither Grant nor I could stand.

Would the doctors morally, ethically have to keep Ben alive, no matter what his condition, as long as there was a drug or a machine that could keep his body going?

"That depends on you," Judie Lea said, answering our question while Ben was still asleep. Judie was leading us through territory that was completely new, guiding us without making our decisions for us.

"We don't want to keep him alive unnaturally, I mean . . . if it is his time to go," Grant said.

"How can we know when it is his time to die, Grant?" Judie said. "Doctors can't decide that. I guess nobody can, really. But the hospital has certain procedures . . . There is a paper you can sign. If you want to."

"A paper?" I asked.

"It calls for no 'drastic measures' to be taken to keep a critically ill patient alive," she said.

Judie reassured us that, were we to sign the papers, Ben would be kept comfortable. He would be given food and water and pain medication. But no "drastic measures" would be taken to keep him alive artificially.

Grant and I talked it over. It didn't take long, because we were of one mind about this. We signed the papers.

Ben was on his own now. If it was time for him to die, we would not stop him. But, as I was signing that document, never had I hoped more fervently that he would live. That his time had not come.

*   *   *

Ben slept for two full days. On the third morning, he opened his eyes. Grant and I looked at each other with immense relief. He was alive. Groggy, but alive. Though Grant and I and Beau were traumatized by that seizure, Ben remembered nothing of it.

And once again, he began fighting to get better. Within a few days, it was as if nothing had happened. And by the end of the week he was, if anything, feistier after his long rest.

The nurses came in to put the dreaded tube back down his throat that they had to remove during the seizure. And he said no. Pleasantly, but firmly. And surprisingly maturely.

"I want to talk to Dr. Glader first," he said. He wasn't being petulant. He was just a patient asking to see his doctor. And Ben knew enough about hospitals by now to understand that the nurse couldn't make the decision. And he didn't want to bother with an intern. He wanted the man in charge.

Dr. Glader came in that afternoon, and Ben told him he felt he had given the tube several weeks to work, and it only made him feel worse instead of better. Now he wanted to try it his way, without the tube. He vomited so often anyway that the gastric juices the tube was supposed to remove came up on their own, he said.

Dr. Glader looked over at me with something akin to an

arched eyebrow. I just smiled. I had been in discussions like this before with Ben. He could be very convincing when he had made up his mind about something, and there was usually a good reason for it. And he had definitely made his mind up about the tube.

"Okay, Ben. I guess you got me. Let's try it your way."

"All right!"

Ben beamed. It was a small moment of self-assertion, but one that helped him reestablish a little control over his life. He hadn't had a lot of that since he'd been back in the hospital this time.

The following week, Grant's father brought Ben's cousins Brett and Joey up for a visit. They bounded in the door in jeans and sneakers and Grampa was right behind them. Ben gave them a great big smile as soon as the door opened. Nobody could bolster his spirits like his cousins.

"Look what we brought you, Ben!" Brett said.

Joey handed Ben a little block of wood, a piece of plain pine about seven inches long and three inches wide. Ben turned it over in his hands. Clearly the cousins were excited about it, but he didn't have the slightest idea why.

"It's for your Pinewood Derby race, Benjamin," Grampa explained. "Ever hear about that in your Cub Scout pack?"

Ben shook his head. He hadn't been to a meeting in so long.

"It's a race. A *big* race," Joey said. "You get this block of wood and then you make it into a car. And then you race it and see who wins. You get medals and everything."

"You mean you get to design your own car . . . anything you want?"

"Yeah! We brought ours too," Brett said. "We can do it together."

"Rad!" Ben exclaimed.

So, Ben and his Grampa and the cousins set up shop right there in the hospital. They pored over pictures of cars in magazines and studied the car models Ben had made since he'd been in the hospital. They discussed the virtues of fins and wind scoops and other things I'd never heard of.

Brett and Joey drew their designs directly onto the wood. But Ben carefully laid his out on paper first. He wanted every detail just so. He drew the car from different angles so he could tell what it would look like when it was done. What he designed was something futuristic, sleek, and high tech, very low in front and rising in the back with a high, curving tail.

Finally he transferred his design to the block of wood.

The other boys were already busy at work carving out their cars when Grampa Oyler got out his prized pocketknife for Ben.

"Can you manage, Benjamin?"

Ben took hold of the heavy knife and gave it a try.

But even though the wood was soft, he didn't have enough strength to carve it.

"Want some help?" Grampa asked.

Ben looked up and smiled.

"Sure."

For a while, Grampa guided Ben's hands. But ultimately, Grampa had to do much of the carving himself.

By the end of the day, there were pine shavings strewn all over the room. And there were three new race cars ready to be painted.

"I want mine metallic red!" Joey said.

"I want mine silver with a black racing stripe," Brett said.

"Grampa, do I have to paint mine?" Ben asked.

"No, I don't think so, Benjamin," he said. "Don't you want to?"

"No, I think I just want to whitewash it like the birdhouse I made once with Grampa Ralph so the wood can show through."

The next weekend there were preliminary trials for the upcoming derby, and we arranged to take Ben home to see how his little car would perform.

But I found myself wishing later that we'd never gone. Ben's car came in last. Dead last. And the brief moments of happiness that the car and the cousins' visit had brought seemed to vanish into thin air.

❋   ❋   ❋

When we got back to the hospital, Ben was very low. What he needed—more than anything—was a friend.

But friends weren't easy to come by for a boy with AIDS. Even in a hospital, parents of other children were afraid to have their children spend too much time with Ben. One day he went out to the courtyard at exactly 3:55 P.M. to wait for another little patient he had met. They had agreed to meet at 4:00 P.M. But five minutes passed, and then ten, and then thirty. Finally, after an hour, when it was getting dark, Ben gave up and went back inside.

Then one day, a man and a woman we had never met stopped by to visit Ben. They were from a group called the Make-a-Wish Foundation, which grants the last wishes of children with fatal diseases.

"If you could have anything you wanted, anything at all, Ben, what would it be?" the lady asked.

He thought for a while.

"A race-car set!" he said.

But the people from the foundation were used to granting far bigger wishes than fifty-dollar race-car sets. They summoned me into the hall and suggested Ben ask for something more, a trip maybe. But Ben was in no shape to travel. Not now. So I suggested a shopping spree at Toys-R-Us. That way Ben could get his race-car set. And other things as well.

Just looking forward to the toy spree lifted Ben's spirits. He made a list of toys he wanted. But when I took a look at it, I noticed almost everything was for Beau and Aber.

When the day came for the shopping trip, Ben turned down a wheelchair. He wanted to walk up and down the aisles on his own.

By the time he was done, I looked at the jumbled array of toys at the checkout counter: some toy guns, a baseball glove, a robot, and the most special thing of all, an electric jeep with two seats.

"You can actually ride in it, Mom!" Ben said.

The days that followed were difficult for Ben. He was too weak to be able to do many of the things he had been doing a few months before, but not so much in pain that he didn't really long to get out to play.

That's when Jaap Suermondt entered Ben's life—all our lives, really.

I first saw Jaap when I walked into Ben's room one afternoon. And there he was, a young blond Stanford student, a hospital volunteer, sitting in the corner reading while Ben was engrossed in his cartoon.

I kissed Ben, and gave him Danny to hold. Then Jaap politely stood up—he was very tall, six feet five inches. He said he was Dutch, and his name was pronounced "Yop." He had come to Stanford to study. His father was a pediatrician in Holland, so Jaap was familiar with hospitals.

I liked Jaap instantly. He had just a slight accent and a formal way of speaking that indicated respect.

After talking to him, I knew why we hadn't seen any volunteers before. Hospital volunteers were allowed to choose the patients they wanted to spend time with, but they were encouraged to circulate, not spend too much time with any one patient. Jaap told me they had been warned that the little boy in Room 205 had AIDS and so no one had volunteered to visit Ben. That is, no one until Jaap.

Jaap admitted to me that he had his own reservations, since

the staff had been so adamant about the precautions that needed to be taken in working with an AIDS patient. He was understandably concerned but, nonetheless, a little embarrassed to admit it.

The thing that dissipated his fears, he told me, was when he saw me hand Danny to Ben.

Ben was a little leery of Jaap at first. Interns about Jaap's age were constantly coming in to study him, and he was tired of being observed by people who cared only about his disease. And though he wanted a new friend, he had been disappointed there too. I don't think he wanted to be disappointed again.

Ben tried to test Jaap before letting him into his life.

"I've got AIDS," Ben told him on the second or third day he was there.

"I know. They told me," Jaap said. "Are you feeling all right now?"

"Right now? Okay. But I'm gonna die, you know."

"Ben, don't talk like that!"

"Why not?"

"Well, just don't, that's all," Jaap said.

Ben changed the subject.

Little by little, Ben came to trust Jaap. The hospital staff overlooked the rule about volunteers becoming attached to individual patients, and Ben and Jaap became a team. One tall, gangly, and blond. The other, a puffy-cheeked little boy with big brown eyes who barely came up to Jaap's waist.

As they got to know each other, Jaap would come by every day to do his homework, just sitting by Ben. The two of them would go on outings sometimes, for a short walk, or to the toy store, or to choose a movie to rent from the video store.

❀   ❀   ❀

Beau turned seven that April. It was a Sunday. I remember walking into Ben's room, and Ben was up, at the door, when I went in. He quickly closed the door behind me before Beau and Aber could come in.

"Can you get a big bow, Mom?" he asked. "And make sure Beau doesn't come in. Okay? Or Aber either, 'cause he'll tell. Promise?"

I turned and saw what looked like a machine gun mounted on his bed.

"What on earth is that?"

"Rambo squirt gun, battery powered."

"Gee, Ben, I don't think I've ever seen a squirt gun quite like that before."

"It's for Beau, Mom. For his birthday. Think he'll like it?"

"He'll love it. Where in the world did you get it?"

"Talked the nurse out of it. The one that's got the keys to the secret closet where they keep all the toys people give to the hospital. What d'ya think?"

"Oh, I think Beau will be very happy."

When Beau finally was allowed back into Ben's room that afternoon, he was, in fact, thrilled. "Rad!" he exclaimed when he saw the squirt gun. That was the biggest compliment in his vocabulary. Ben had it preloaded, and he showed Beau how to aim it, just so, out the window. Clearly, he had practiced up a little himself.

We all cheered.

"Good shot, Beau!" Ben shouted.

And from the nurses' station down the hall, we heard Dr. Glader's voice.

"Hey, Ben! Keep it down in there, okay?"

We all stopped for a minute and looked at each other like children caught talking in class. Then Ben burst out laughing. He had a different laugh now than he used to. But it was back, I thought. His laugh was back.

Beau couldn't take his eyes off his Rambo squirt gun.

"Thank you, Ben," Beau said. "That's my best birthday present ever."

And he reached out and hugged Ben.

There was something very special about that ordinary little scene. We were enjoying ourselves, enjoying each other, under the worst possible circumstances. Maybe Grant and I had had it wrong those first few months after Ben's diagnosis, when we had been trying to follow routine to make life look as if nothing had changed.

Things *had* changed. And one of the major changes was that we didn't have a routine to follow. There was a certain freedom in that. Living each day as it came and loving each other more openly than we ever had before. There weren't any schedules, or even any habits, that told us we weren't supposed to talk about the things that mattered.

*   *   *

It was realizations like that that helped me get through the days. Though the seizure had left Ben physically weaker, he was unaffected mentally by that awful ordeal. But I don't think Grant and I ever really got over it.

I was afraid to sleep. It was almost as if I were expecting to be wakened to hear that Ben had had another seizure. I was afraid to leave Ben's room, for fear that once I got down the hall, I would hear that voice paging "Stat, Room 205."

Grant went back to work. But he was so worried, so isolated from our family that he had trouble concentrating. And I was worried about him. He even looked bad. One weekend when he came up, Judie Lea took one look at him and told us point-blank we ought to try to get away.

I knew she was right. We could use some time away from the hospital. Away from sickness. Away from the constant fear. But how? When? There didn't seem to be a way.

Then, Ben said to me one day, "Mom, do you think Grampa Ralph would take a look at my derby car? Maybe he could figure out what to do to make it faster."

"We could ask him, but I don't know when Grampa and Gramma might be coming up, Ben. Los Angeles is a long drive, you know."

"Well, maybe you can take it to him."

"Who's going to stay here with you?"

"Jaap. Jaap can take care of me, can't you, Jaap?" he asked, turning to Jaap, who was doing his homework in the corner of Ben's room.

"Sure. Ben and I'll have a great time," he said.

"Oh, please, Mom," Ben begged. It was as if he too knew we needed the time away.

"Okay, I'll call Grampa Ralph," I said.

Ralph had raised three sons of his own. He had been a Cub Scout leader himself. He'd know what to do. If anyone could work magic with one little Pinewood Derby car, it was Ralph.

"Bring it on down, we'll give it a try," Ralph told Grant when he called him to say how disappointed Ben was about the car's performance. "It's been twenty years since I tried my hand at a Pinewood Derby car, Grant. I'll have to do a little brushing up on the rules. But I think we can fix it up a little."

Leave it to Ralph. And to my mother, who immediately volunteered to take Beau and Aber for a few days while Grant, Danny, and I went to San Diego, to stay at Torrey Pines, where Grant and I had spent wonderful times together on the golf course before we were married.

Grant played golf for the first time since Ben had gotten sick. He got up at 4:00 A.M. each day to sign up to play early in the day at the popular public course. Then he'd come back and get a little more sleep until it was time to tee off.

After the second night of Danny keeping me up, Grant took him along in the stroller so I could get some rest. When he came back, I noticed something dangling down to the back of his knees. Something that looked a little like a tail on a kite.

"What's that you're dragging around behind you?" I asked.

He fumbled around in the dark.

I could almost see his face reddening.

He held up my nursing bra.

"Oh, no, you mean I've been walking around with this thing dangling behind me?"

I just burst out laughing.

"I can see it now, all those old-timers waiting around the pro shop to sign up to play. And then up walks this young guy pushing a stroller with a six-month-old baby in it and a nursing bra hanging out of the back of his pants! They must have gotten a real hoot out of that after you left!"

Then Grant laughed too. We both did. And it felt so good, we laughed some more. Laughed and laughed until we felt our sides were going to split. I had never realized how regenerating it is to laugh.

"That's what you get for getting up at four in the morning and dressing in the dark," I said.

"And this is what you get for leaving your bra on the same chair with my pants," he said, flopping down on the bed and kissing me between laughs.

And then he kissed me some more. And then it was as if we both remembered we were together in the same city, in the same bed for the first time in ages. And we didn't have a single place we had to go or a single thing we had to do.

And Danny, bless his little heart, slept.

※　　※　　※

I realized while we were gone how desperately Grant and I needed those few days away. But now we were anxious to get back, anxious to see our little boy. There was only one stop we had to make on our way back up . . .

Beau and Aber came running out to meet us when the white van drove up to the curb of my mom's house, and four little arms wrapped themselves around me as soon as I stepped out of the car.

While I played with Beau and Aber and caught up with my mom, Grant and Ralph headed out to his workshop to work on the Pinewood Derby car.

First they sanded the axles and the wheels of the little car with the finest-grade sandpaper they could find. Then Ralph figured out a way to tilt the wheels so they wouldn't rub up against the body of the car when it rolled.

Ralph brought to bear all his experience from the Pinewood Derby races his sons had competed in years before. He drilled a half-inch hole in the underbelly of the car and set it upside down on a postage scale. Then he and Grant dropped BBs into the hole, one by one, until the car weighed the legal limit. Exactly five ounces, no more, no less. He glued a strip of wood over the hole, and they were ready to give it a try.

We all went out to the wood shop for the test run—Mom and Beau and Aber and me. Ralph had propped a board up against a chair to simulate the racetrack in the derby. Then he placed it at the high end, and let it go. The little whitewashed race car took off with a life all its own, and didn't stop until it hit the wall on the other side of the room.

"Wowww, Grampa!" Beau said.

Ralph just took a deep breath and smiled.

* * *

It was a shock to get back to the hospital and to see everything with fresh eyes. Everything was the same, only worse, because we had had a chance to step outside and remember what it was like in the world outside the hospital.

Ben was thrilled with what Grampa Ralph had done to his Pinewood Derby car. Now it was fast. Really fast. I told the nurses we'd have to be sure to leave by noon on Saturday at the latest so we could get home, set up Ben's equipment, and be at the races by 7:00 P.M. Grant was going to drive up Friday night when he finished work.

But at 11:00 P.M. Friday he still hadn't arrived. And I began to worry. Finally the phone rang at the Ronald Mc-Donald House.

It was Grant. His voice was tense.

"I don't want you to worry, Chris. I'm okay."

I panicked.

"Grant, what happened? Where are you?"

"I'm in Carmel. I think I had a heart attack when I was finishing up the Guzmans' kitchen."

"A WHAT?"

He told me how he had been dusting off grout on the kitchen he'd just tiled when he remembered he had to get to the hardware store by 9:00 P.M. to buy something to hook up the sink. So he had dropped what he was doing, run to the store, and eaten a candy bar on the way back because he hadn't had anything since breakfast. He started furiously removing the grout from the tile because it was drying fast.

"Then it just hit me," he said. "I just felt this pain go down my arm, and couldn't breathe, and I almost fell over."

"Did you go to the doctor?"

"I'm waiting for Dr. Rasband to come over now. I'll call you as soon as he gets here. I just didn't want you to worry."

Not worry?

I was too scared to move. I just lay there in bed in the dark imagining the worst, because I knew now that the worst could happen. Grant was only thirty-one years old. But people that young do die of heart attacks. And he had been working unbelievable hours under unbelievable stress.

Nothing could happen to Grant. I loved him too much. I needed him too much. He was my pillar of strength, the only person I really could turn to in the midst of Ben's illness. What would we do if he got sick? What would we ever do without him?

I just lay there, terrified, waiting for the telephone to ring. Waiting for him to call back and say he was okay.

When he finally did, the news was good. Dr. Rasband checked him over and found no sign of a heart attack. He just said Grant had been working too hard. I finally got to sleep.

No longer scared. Just worried. Somehow we had to find a way to ease the stress on Grant. But I didn't see how to make the stress go away.

I needed to see him. I needed to know for myself that Grant was all right. I knew what a terrible strain he had been under, but I guess I had been so caught up in trying to take care of Ben and the other boys that I didn't want to see it. I needed Grant to be strong and dependable and . . . there, just there. I always needed for Grant to be there. I couldn't think of something being wrong with Grant because I couldn't stand for one more thing to be wrong.

When Grant drove up the next morning, I was so glad to see him. At first I just hugged him, holding on as tight as I could. Then I stared at him, studying his face to make sure he was okay. He looked fine. Grant was so handsome, so healthy-looking. He still had that strong body of a college athlete and that boy-next-door sort of face.

"Are you sure you're all right?" I asked.

"The doctor said I'm fine. Really. I'm okay."

"You'd tell me, right?"

"Of course I would. You know I would. It's just stress. Come on. We gotta get going."

With that, he just brushed off the incident of the night before as if it were nothing. Maybe it was. Maybe I was worrying too much. Maybe all I knew how to do anymore was worry. Anyway, Grant said he was okay and I believed him. I wanted to believe him.

We hurriedly packed the van and got Ben ready to go

home so he could participate in the Pinewood Derby that night.

Leaving the hospital always felt like a triumph. But this time in particular, we were glad to be going home. Ben needed constant home nursing care now, but the public agency that had funded his nursing before, the California Children's Society, had run out of money. It had taken three weeks and a lot of effort on the part of the hospital staff to help us arrange home nursing care under Medi-Cal. But finally all the preparations were made.

Just checking out of the hospital was increasingly time-consuming now. Ben had so many medications and pieces of equipment that we were late taking off. Then we hit traffic. It was close to 6:00 P.M. before we got home and Ben said he was tired, he had to take a nap. The Pinewood Derby was at seven.

Beau stood and watched as I tried to wake Ben about 6:45, but he couldn't even get out of bed.

"I can't, Mom," he mumbled.

Beau knew how excited Ben had been about the race. He knew how badly he would feel if he missed it. He and Aber were excited too. They were all ready to go cheer their big brother on.

"Ben, how about if I race it for you?" Beau asked.

"That would be great, Beau . . ." Ben barely got the words out and fell back asleep.

So, I stayed home with Ben while Grant and Aber went out to watch Beau race with the big boys. They got there late, so Beau missed the preliminary heats and had to race the winner of Ben's whole troop.

Beau lined Ben's car up at the top of the ramp along with the other boy's winning car, and together they let go to see whose reached the finish line first.

Ben's car won by a mile. Then Beau raced the winner of the older Boy Scout division.

Beau won the grand prize. Or rather, as Beau put it, Ben won the grand prize.

"You won, Ben! You won!" Beau shouted as soon as he got in the front door. "You won the whole thing!"

8

"Daddy Smashed the Crib!"

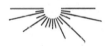

I DON'T KNOW whose triumph was the greatest in that Pinewood Derby, Ben's or Beau's.

For weeks afterward, every detail of every race was told and retold. Ben couldn't hear it enough. It was a constant source of joy for him. A special kind of victory in his life, when victories were hard to come by.

But for Beau, winning the derby meant doing something for Ben. Something that Ben couldn't do for himself and something that earned Ben's respect. It's hard sometimes for little brothers to shine in a big brother's eyes, but this time Beau was truly shining. And nothing meant as much to Beau as praise from Ben.

In an odd sort of way, that Pinewood Derby was an opportunity we never could have come up with if we had tried. I knew in my heart that that experience was something Beau and Ben would both remember forever. It was truly a gift they had given each other.

❈   ❈   ❈

I don't remember much about the next two weeks except that Ben's pain got worse.

But I do remember May 2. That was the night that Ben had another seizure.

This time I was there when it happened. It started at exactly 11:00 P.M., when the nursing shift changed, so two nurses were on hand. They administered the emergency seizure medication that we had taped to Ben's bedroom wall. Grant and I held Ben down and I could feel the convulsions wrack Ben's body over and over and over again.

For me, it was more terrifying than the first. Not because the seizure was worse; it was clearly milder. But because this time Ben was awake when it started. This time he would remember it happening. And I knew he would be afraid.

I sat on the edge of his bed for an hour or two that night, just looking at his sleeping face.

It had been almost a year now since Ben had been diagnosed as having AIDS. Fifty-one weeks of constant vomiting, constant diarrhea, and of coughing and infections and pains that had run at will through his forty-five-pound body. And he had taken it all virtually without complaint.

But how much more could he take? How many more "symptoms" would he have to accumulate?

The doctor's words came back to me. "Eighty-five percent are dead within a year. Eighty-five percent."

I was so torn, so confused. There were only two things I wanted: for Ben to live, and for Ben not to have to suffer anymore.

Now it no longer seemed possible to have both.

When we took Ben back to the hospital the next day, the

doctors put him on morphine. Now Ben was so drugged he didn't recognize us most of the time. We'd try to talk to him and his eyes would swim to the back of his head.

A nurse told us that things were fine, that he was being "regulated" on pain medicine. And as long as he was "arousable," everything was all right.

But everything wasn't all right. Grant and I would walk in in the morning and Ben would try to talk and his speech would be so slurred we couldn't understand a word. Then he'd fall back into a stupor.

On the third day, we tried to shake him awake.

"Ben? Ben? Can you understand what I'm saying to you?" Grant asked.

"Yeah . . . ," and his eyes would roll back in his head.

"Benny, listen to me, honey," I said. "Don't you want to see Danny and play with Beau and Aber?" He didn't answer.

"You don't want to keep on living like this, do you?"

"I'mmm fine . . . ," he slurred.

It was no use.

For the first time, Grant and I disagreed with the hospital's approach to Ben's treatment. Was this the way they expected Ben to live whatever remained of the rest of his life? Whether Ben lived another two days or another two years, he should at least be aware he was living them.

Finally, we walked up to the doctor who was treating Ben at the time and told him he had to find another way to relieve Ben's pain. He was surprised at our request. After all, he pointed out, Ben wasn't in pain. We explained to him that the medicine had taken away more than the pain; it had taken away our son. He agreed to bring in a pain specialist to come up with an alternative approach.

After studying Ben's case that afternoon, the specialist proposed a synthetic form of morphine he felt would allow Ben to remain more alert while still alleviating his pain. But, he stressed, Ben himself would be the key to making this new plan work. Everything depended on his ability to communicate with the nurses, telling them as precisely as he could just how bad his pain was, so they would know exactly how much medicine to give him. That way, Ben would never be either undermedicated or overmedicated. And, if all went right, they would be able to control the pain.

That night the nurses began taking Ben off the morphine. Grant came in and kissed his groggy son good night. He had to drive back to Carmel . . . again. Would I ever get used to these partings? It seemed to get harder and harder every time I walked Grant out to the parking lot and watched his pickup drive off in the dark.

That night when I climbed into bed at the Ronald McDonald House, I found a note on my pillow from Grant:

Dear Chris,

Just a short note to tell you that I adore you. I want you to know how much I've missed you these past weeks and months. Especially when I was home. There is not a thing in our home that does not make me think of you. As I drive up I see the flowers you have planted in our neat yard. The inside is made by and chosen by you. You bring such beauty and cleanliness and happiness to our home.

If you can believe it, I even missed looking over at your beautiful face sleeping in the car and holding your hand.

You sure make me happy. You're going to be a tough act to follow when our boys marry. I'm sure they will handle it well, though.

You are so dear to me. All five of you are. I have thought about you every moment you were away and prayed for us all to be together again.

> Love,
> G.O.

I cried—but this time for joy—and then fell asleep.

I woke up the next morning with new determination. I was going to get Ben out of bed. Not just out of bed, but out-of-doors. Out into the sunshine and fresh air. Maybe that would help clear the fog that enveloped him.

It was a pleasant spring day and we could hear the birds chirping as we sat down next to each other in the courtyard. We just sat there for a while looking at the grass and the sky.

"I'm afraid it'll hurt, Mom," he said.

"We'll get you some different medicine, Ben."

"I mean when I die, Mom."

I looked at Ben and my heart stood still. There was total acceptance written on his face. No panic. No fear. None of the denial and confusion I felt in my own heart. Just something that said: I knew this was going to happen and I can handle it, I'm ready, but I just need a little help.

Even then, I wanted to tell him he was wrong, that he wasn't going to die. Even then, my instinct was to tell him everything would be all right.

Only I couldn't, because that wasn't quite the truth. Ben needed me to be honest, and not afraid. That was what he needed from me to get through this.

"Ben, honey, are you afraid of dying?"

Ben shook his head.

"No, Mom. I'm just afraid it's gonna hurt."

"Oh, Benny, I can understand that, because you've been through so much. But it won't hurt. I promise. I'll make sure you get whatever medicine you need to take away the pain. And we can start praying that the Holy Ghost will give you special comfort right now, okay?"

He nodded. But I could tell he was still afraid . . . a little.

"Does it hurt now?"

"Just a little. Not very much."

"On a scale of one to ten, with ten being the worst, how bad would you say the pain is right now?"

He thought for a minute.

"It's okay, Mom. It's just a two."

"I tell you what, Ben. I've been talking a lot with the nurses. And they say that if you can rate the pain for them, from one to ten, then they'll give you whatever medicine you need to make you feel better. How does that sound?"

"Okay, Mom."

"Oh, Benny, I wish I could change places with you. I've

wished that so many times, so you wouldn't have to go through all this."

"I know, Mom. But I'd never let you do that anyway."

I just looked at him. I was trying so hard not to cry, but the tears came anyway. I wanted so badly to be brave for Ben. And he was the one who was being brave for me.

Then Ben asked me a favor, a favor I later thought of as one he did more for me than for himself.

"Will you rock me like you used to when I was little?"

He put his arms around my neck and I cradled him in my arms.

I don't know how long we sat there on that bench. Just rocking back and forth.

I just remember the joy and the warmth of holding my son in my arms. I thought about all the hours I had rocked him as a baby. My first-born. And I wanted that moment to last forever.

❧   ❧   ❧

Early in June, Grant had another attack. He felt he was choking and could not breathe. His heart was palpitating, and he felt he was going to lose consciousness. He ended up in a hospital emergency room.

The doctor who treated him confirmed Dr. Rasband's initial diagnosis. Grant had had another "stress attack." He suggested Grant see a psychologist, take some time off from work, and try to eliminate the stress in his life.

This time I really started to worry. Grant had brushed the first incident off all too lightly. Obviously, there was something really wrong and I didn't know what to do about it. I felt helpless.

There was no way we could eliminate the stress in his life. How could we? There was stress everywhere. In my life and in his.

I urged Grant to stop working and told him we'd manage somehow. He did slow down, but he couldn't quit completely because of our financial needs and because of work commitments he had made. The most he could do was take a sedative if he felt another attack coming on and lie down.

Before, Grant and I had always been able to lean on each other. We had always been able to shift our weight and support each other. When he was down, I would bolster him up again. When I felt lost and defeated, he would be strong for me.

Now there was no strength left in either of us. There was no place to lean. Keeping our family going and taking care of Ben and worrying about losing him had taken all the strength either of us had.

It seemed lonely. As though we each had to fend for ourselves. Grant knew I had all I could handle. And I knew I couldn't burden him.

To protect Grant's health, I began keeping the small crises in our lives to myself. Beau's struggle to come to grips with the loss of his big brother. Arguments between Beau and Aber. Household problems.

Beau would want to talk at night, just when I was the most exhausted and was trying to settle Aber and the baby down for the night. One night, I was finally getting Danny to sleep when Aber began bouncing from bed to bed. I felt as though I hadn't slept at all the night before because of Danny, and Beau could see I was just at my wits' end.

Just when I thought I couldn't take another minute of horseplay, Beau pulled Aber down with him under the covers.

"I'm tired," Beau announced. "Go to sleep, Aber."

"I'm tired, too," Aber parroted. "Go to sleep, Mommy."

"Good night, boys," I said, gratefully. I didn't understand Beau's sudden fatigue, but I wasn't about to question it.

I was just about asleep when I heard Beau whisper in the dark.

"We sure fooled Aber, didn't we, Mom?"

I laughed in spite of my exhaustion. "Yes, Beau. We sure did. Thanks for thinking of me. You're a good big brother to Aber. Good night, now."

The quiet lasted maybe ten seconds.

"Mom?"

"Yes?"

"Aber's scared, Mom."

"Why? What's he scared of?"

"He's scared 'cause he's afraid Ben's gonna die."

I could hear Beau sniffling in the dark, trying not to let on he was crying. I moved over to his bed and held him. He was such a sturdy little guy, the kind of boy who would grow up one day to be so strong on the outside that you wouldn't guess how sensitive he was on the inside.

"It's all right to cry, Beau. I cry too. We don't know what's going to happen to Ben. But do you remember what we talked about? About how dying isn't something you should be scared of? And about how we'll all be together again in heaven? Can you remember to tell that to Aber?"

"Yeah. But Mom, I don't want Ben to die, too. I really, really don't want Ben to die. I just want him to stay here with us."

"I know, honey. I know."

* * *

It wasn't until June that home nursing was arranged so Ben could leave the hospital. His care was so complicated now that there were three typed pages just listing his medications. We brought Jaap home with us for a few days before he returned to Holland for the summer.

During that short visit, Ben showed Jaap all his favorite Carmel places. Oscar Hossenfellder's merry-go-round. The park with the giant slide, which he insisted Jaap try out. The hill where he'd ridden his bicycle to school with Beau. The ugly knots of flower bulbs that had now produced long green leaves.

"I hope I see you again," Jaap said to Ben when we took him to the plane. It was as close as Jaap ever came, I think, to admitting in words to Ben that he knew he was dying.

"You will," Ben said.

*   *   *

Perhaps the one thing that had sustained Grant and me through that year was the solid foundation of our marriage. Grant had always been a source of strength to me. I depended on him so much. And suddenly it was as if he wasn't there.

If he felt a stress attack coming on, he'd have to take a sedative and lie down. And it scared me every time I saw him starting to hyperventilate and having a hard time breathing.

I didn't want to tell him about problems because I didn't want to add more stress to his life. But I needed him now. I had a lot of stress too. But I couldn't take a sedative and lie down. I just couldn't. Somehow I had to keep going. And one of the things that had always kept me going was just knowing Grant was there. Now, I had no place to lean. No Grant to tell me everything would be okay. No Grant to tell me we would get through this. No Grant to help me. To reassure me.

I began to grow resentful, to feel he'd quit on me. Only I couldn't talk to him about it, because that would have only brought on another attack. So I began to withdraw.

I began to feel that our lives were on parallel courses, mirroring each other but never touching. It was all the more unbearable because we had never been like that before. Whatever had happened, we could always talk.

I didn't like what our lives had become. Or the distance between us. I had read somewhere about how many couples get divorces over the loss of a child, how they can't survive the pain and the grief. That couldn't happen to us. Not to Grant and me. We had gotten married forever. Whatever problems we had, they were our problems. Not Grant's. Not mine. And we had to get through them together.

Late one afternoon I came home with the baby, and Beau and Aber came running up to me in tears. "Daddy smashed the crib!" Aber said.

They led me into the house and showed me Danny's crib. There was a hole the size of a fist right through the headboard, just above the little pastel lambs. My stomach sank, seeing the splintered crib that had been Grant's as a baby. I couldn't make sense of what had happened. Grant had done this? Grant Oyler? Never had I seen him do anything like this before. It just wasn't like him.

I tried to calm the boys. I told them Daddy hadn't been feeling like himself lately because he'd been working so hard. When they had quieted down and were playing, I put Danny down for a nap at the far end of the crib, and went into the bedroom. Grant was just sitting there on the edge of the bed with his head in his hands.

"Grant, what happened?"

"I don't know."

He just sat there. Silent.

"You don't know how you smashed the crib?"

"Yes . . . no. I mean I don't know why. I don't know what

came over me. The boys were arguing, and they wouldn't calm down and I, I . . . I just lost control and I hit the crib. It was the closest thing I could find. I'm sorry. I feel awful. Can't we put a little wooden cloud over the hole?"

The little scene on the crib was so small, so dainty. I could just imagine this giant wooden cloud glued over these little tiny lambs. The idea was so . . . so Grant. Thinking he could just cover something up and pretend it would go away.

"Forget the crib, Grant. What's done is done. It's you I'm worried about. You and me and the boys. We need you, Grant. I need you. More than I've ever needed you in my life. And I can't depend on you for anything anymore. I can't even get you to talk about it."

"How can I talk to you about it when you're so mad at me all the time?"

"Don't you think I have a right to be mad when you go off and have your stress attacks and leave me with everything? Everything. Ben, the boys, the baby, the house? You never used to be like this, Grant. You were always there whenever I needed you."

"Everybody needs me. Don't you understand that, Chris? Everybody is depending on me and I keep letting everybody down. When I'm at work, I feel guilty because I should be with you and Ben. I want to be with you, but I can't. And when the weekend comes and I'm with you, I feel guilty because I need to be working. I'm always behind schedule. I never finish a job on time anymore and people are always mad at me.

"I'm letting everybody down. You. Ben. Clients. Beau and Aber. Everybody. I can never, ever be where I want to be and need to be at the same time anymore. Never.

"I have always tried to be there for you. I have. But now I need you and you're not there. Why? Why can't you be there for me now . . . when I need you?"

Grant's words stung. He was right. I wasn't being fair. Or understanding. But Grant? Did Grant really need me for emotional support the way I needed him? He had always been the one who was strong.

"I wanted to help, Grant. I tried. I tried to talk. I tried to get you to face this. To do what the doctor told you to do. To slow down on work and go see that psychologist. But you won't do it. You won't talk to me about it and you won't talk to the psychologist. You're just pretending it will go away. Well, it won't go away."

Grant looked up at me with tears in his eyes.

"I'm sorry," I said. "But what made you think I had anything left to give? My oldest son is dying and I've got two other little boys and all their emotional needs to deal with, and a new baby. Maybe I'm all given out. It's not the fact that you have the stress attacks that bothers me. It's the fact that you won't face up to it and try to get better."

"Maybe I don't want to face up to it. Okay? Maybe I can't . . . maybe I don't know how. I don't even understand what's wrong. The only thing the doctor says is to take a pill whenever I feel one of these attacks coming on. And what's a psychologist supposed to do? The pain is in my chest."

He sat very still.

"I get so scared, Chris. And so mad. Because Ben's in there dying and there's not one single thing I can do about it. Do you know what that does to my insides? Just to think about that? My whole life my dad did everything for us. No matter what went wrong, he'd fix it. And here when my son really, really needs me, Chris . . . Chris, I can't do anything. Not one thing."

He made a fist with his right hand and started to slam it into the open palm of his left hand, then he just stopped in midair, and leaned over and held me and broke down and cried. I held him as tightly as I could and I cried with him.

"No matter how much we hurt now, we can't hurt each other, Grant. Not anymore. Ben needs us, both of us. We need to love him and we need to love each other."

*　　*　　*

I don't think it was until that day that Grant really stopped counting on a miracle to make Ben better. He had believed in that miracle for so long. It had sustained him through trying hours alone, far away from his family. I had long since given up on that kind of a miracle. . . . That didn't mean Grant's faith was stronger than mine. And it didn't mean that I was any more realistic than he was.

We were just two different people in love with the same little boy, trying to do everything we could for him, each in our own way. There was no right way to cope with the fact that our child was dying. And there was no wrong way. There was only Grant's way and mine.

But now it was time to set aside our differences. Time to stop thinking of our own pain, and time to focus on our son. Ben had a new journey ahead of him. One we ourselves had heard about, but never taken.

9

"They Usually See a Light"

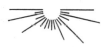

I HAD JUST GOTTEN OUT OF THE SHOWER the next morning when I heard Beau and Aber cheering outside.

"C'mon, Ben!"

"You can do it, Ben!"

I wiped away the steam from the bathroom window and looked out into the backyard. There was Ben in his baggy jeans and suspenders with a baseball bat in his hands.

Grant had a softball in his hand and was standing in front of him, maybe only five or six feet away. Then he began pitching the ball to Ben. Slowly, deliberately. Each time, Ben would swing unsteadily and miss. Then Grant would walk up, get the ball, and start all over again. "That's right, Ben. Hold the bat up. Are you sure you're not too tired? Okay then. Try to swing straight, don't chop wood. Come on, you can do it, Ben."

It was excruciating to watch, this father and son trying so hard to make up for a lifetime.

That deal we'd made on the golf course before we were married about me raising the children until they were twelve, and then Grant taking over. Well, Grant never got his turn with Ben.

Ben would have started Little League this year, but Grant wouldn't ever get a chance to cheer Ben on at a game now.

He wouldn't ever find out whether that chubby little boy would grow up to beat his dad on the golf course.

He wouldn't get a chance to shepherd Ben through adolescence or to stand and applaud as he got his high school diploma . . . or to ever know his son as a man.

What would you have looked like all grown up, Ben?

When you were a baby, I had this picture in my mind of you as a college freshman home for Christmas vacation. You'd bound up the walk, and drop your bags by the door, and give me a big hug and kiss. And then we'd talk a mile a minute so I could catch up on your new life, full of new friends and new interests.

I had even imagined how it would feel inside, that bittersweet mix of pride and nostalgia when you realize your son is a man.

But Ben's still here with us now. Just outside my window.

Suddenly I heard a sound. A familiar sound—the soft but solid whack of wood striking the leather of a worn softball. I looked out just in time to see the ball go flying across the grass and the boys cheering and Grant running up to his son and whirling him high into the air.

Ben was smiling. Exhilarated, triumphant.

"You did it, Ben!" Grant said.

"Way to go, Ben!" Beau shouted.

❈   ❈   ❈

Coming to terms with the brevity of Ben's life was harder for Grant than for me. As short as Ben's life was, I had lived most of it with him. And our times together had been full. But Grant felt cheated.

When he finally went to the psychologist, she suggested a stress-reducing technique. First she had him close his eyes and then imagine being in a beautiful, peaceful place. What came to mind, he said, was a spring meadow in the High Sierras where he had gone hiking with his family years before. And then he imagined his grandfather, his grandmother, and others he loved who had died, sitting beside him.

That small exercise helped Grant do something even more important than reduce the stress in his life. Somehow, it helped him realize that Ben would never be alone. Not in this life or the next. That there were many people who loved Ben and cared about him who would be there for Ben where we couldn't yet go. That after we walked him to the door and let him go through alone there would be loving, familiar out-stretched arms waiting to guide Ben to the other side.

⁂   ⁂   ⁂

There were times when I thought that Ben's death was hardest to understand for Beau.

Beau was too young to accept that death was part of life, and too old not to realize all Ben was going through. Beau had never known a life apart from Ben. He had no past to remember without him. No ability to imagine what life would be like without Ben. No Ben to go to for advice. Or to settle an argument with Aber. Or just to play with.

Ben was not only Beau's best friend, he was his big brother, his ideal. I don't think Beau was ever able to separate Ben from his position as big brother. They were one and the same.

Grant and I witnessed the very moment when I believe Beau finally realized that he was going to lose his big brother. It happened one afternoon when they were playing transformers, those complicated plastic devices that turn from robots into cars or planes and back again.

Then some little argument erupted between them.

"That one's mine," Ben said.

"No, it's not, it's mine," Beau said.

"No, the Gobot's mine. The Autobot's yours," Ben said back.

And he stood up to take it back from Beau. But when he went to grab the toy, he suddenly found he wasn't as tall as Beau anymore, and he wasn't as strong.

And I think Beau realized the same thing at exactly the same time. Ben was older. But Beau was bigger. And for a split second, they just stood there, looking at each other.

Then Beau said quickly, "Here, Ben, you can have it," trying to find a way to take that moment back.

But it was too late, and he knew it.

Beau started to cry. And they just stood there facing each other. Finally, Beau reached out and hugged Ben. And Ben cried too. I couldn't remember the last time I'd seen Ben cry.

Grant and I just watched. There was nothing we could do. Beau was the big brother now. Even before Ben was gone.

That night when I tucked Beau in bed, he asked, "Mom, Ben's going to die soon, isn't he?"

I leaned over and stroked his forehead and said, "Yes, Beau, it could be soon."

He tried not to cry so loud that Ben could hear.

"But Mom, I don't want him to die. Ben's special . . ."

"I know, honey."

"Mom, I wish it was me."

My heart burst just to think how much Beau was hurting inside, how much had been going on inside my little first-grader's mind, how much he had had to think through on his own while Grant and I were so involved with Ben.

"Oh, Beau. Don't say that, honey. You're very, very special too. Daddy and I love you very much."

"But Ben's the big brother."

"That's true, Beau. But you're a big brother too. To Aber and Danny. I know Ben wants you to be a very good big brother to them, just as he has been for you. Do you think you could do that for Ben?"

Beau wasn't the sort to make a commitment and forget about it later. If he agreed to something, he did it. But Beau didn't know if he could do this. He didn't want to take Ben's place. He cried in my arms and shook his head and said again and again that he just didn't want Ben to die.

Then, just before he fell asleep in my arms, he said, "Mom, if I'm the big brother on earth, when we get to heaven, can Ben be the big brother again?"

"I think that's exactly the way Ben would want it, Beau."

❊   ❊   ❊

The next morning, Ben awoke with sores on his lower back, another outbreak of shingles. Shingles were exceptionally painful for him, traveling along the skin above the nerves and sending stabbing pain all over his lower back. Ben had had them in the hospital a few weeks before. But there didn't seem to be much the doctors could do about them then, and now the shingles were back again.

I called Judie Lea. When she said to bring him back to the hospital, I hesitated. I said I'd talk to Grant and let her know. Grant and I talked it over and I called her back.

"We've decided not to bring him up, Judie," I said. "He's too sick. He needs to be home now. We're going to keep our family together."

I expected her to protest. I suppose I wanted her to, because that would have meant there was something else the hospital could do for Ben. But she didn't. There was a brief silence before she answered.

"I understand, Chris. We all do. Just know we're here if you change your mind."

We were on our own now.

As I hung up the phone, I started to think how much of my energy—and my short time with my son—had been taken up on the sheer logistics of fighting this disease. The constant packing and unpacking, the arranging with friends and relatives to take the boys, the scheduling of nurses, the perpetual washing of laundry, the trying to keep house and home together.

That part of this battle was over now. There would be no more long drives to the hospital, no struggling to make that room behind the double isolation doors feel like our home.

Now, we could be together, Ben and Beau and Aber and Danny and Grant and me, together in our own home.

And suddenly I wasn't afraid anymore, not the way I had been that first time we had brought Ben home from the hospital and I felt so alone and scared of the responsibility of taking care of Ben.

I knew what to do. And it was surprisingly easy. All I needed to do was to be Ben's mom. That's all.

I looked out the sliding glass door and saw Ben sitting in the sun on the steps. Beau was trying to get a soggy old tennis ball out of Darcy's mouth to give to Ben to throw again.

"Ben? Judie says we don't have to go back up to the hospital!"

"That's great, Mom!" he said.

* * *

Ben and I spent a lot of time alone together those next few weeks. In the mornings, after a shower, he'd lie down on our bedroom floor in the sun.

It hurt him just to be hugged now. His skin was so sensitive from the shingles, and the shooting pains were so sharp. And his bones were so fragile that he ached all the time.

Sometimes we'd go to the beach to watch the waves crash into the shore, or to spot the seals gallivanting about the rocks.

We'd sit there on the sand and recall special times we had spent in the past. Days at the beach with the cousins, at his Gramma and Grampa Oyler's house in San Clemente. Camping trips we'd taken as a family. Skiing at Park City. Aber's first steps. Beau's first bike ride. Danny's first smile.

It was both heartwarming and heartbreaking to hear Ben recall those times. He described small moments so vividly I could almost imagine we were reliving them. Then I'd turn and see Ben's face, and reality would come back.

Ben demonstrated to me in those quiet times that he would carry only good memories with him of this life. He made me wonder if he was trying to tell me not to look back and wish anything were different. Because he didn't.

There was a peaceful quality about our times together. The noise was gone now. That noise in my ears that sounded like the hum of a million fluorescent lights. The noise I had first heard when Dr. Glader told me Ben had AIDS. It had returned again and again during the past year. But now it was gone.

That hum was the sound of fear. And when I stopped being afraid, it went away. And in its place was a quiet grief. Sad but peaceful.

❧   ❧   ❧

Ben's ninth birthday was June 28.

I remembered Ben's first birthday. How could I forget?

We were at an Oyler family reunion in Lake Tahoe and it was the first birthday of an Oyler grandchild. Grant's dad held Ben in his arms as we helped him blow out the candles. Ben had no idea what the excitement was all about, except that it was for him. And he giggled this contagious little giggle that made all of us laugh.

On Ben's second birthday, he had wanted a Bert 'n' Ernie cake, like the characters from Sesame Street. And I had baked him what he considered the best cake ever made, with gobs of blue and orange frosting. He talked about that cake for months.

Every year after that, for all the boys, we'd have family parties where we'd all play pin-the-tail-on-the-donkey or drop-the-clothespin-in-the-bottle. And somewhere along the line, Ben fell in love with lemon cake with that gooey lemon frosting drizzled on it.

For Ben's ninth birthday, we decided to invite Mom and Ralph up. And, because I knew he would expect it, I made lemon cake and homemade vanilla ice cream to go with it.

When the candles were lit, Grant helped Ben out to the living room.

He walked like an old man now, shuffling forward slowly and haltingly. He leaned slightly to the left, favoring the side that hurt the most. His body had begun to retain water, and his cheeks and eyes and forehead were puffier than ever before. By the time he reached the living room, he was out of breath.

"Happy birthday, Ben!" Aber shouted.

We sang "Happy Birthday," and with our help, Ben blew

out the candles on his cake. He tasted the frosting, gave a spoonful of ice cream to Danny, and asked to go back to bed.

He slept late the next morning.

Mom and Ralph were waiting for Ben to get up to say good-bye. Mom asked Beau and Aber if they wanted to drive down with her for a visit.

"No, thanks, Gramma," Beau said, kissing her good-bye. "I want to stay with Ben."

"Can I go, Mommy, all by myself?" Aber asked, very excitedly.

"Sure, if you'd like to."

Ben listened to the conversation from the sofa. Then his gramma went over to say good-bye.

"I wish I could go with you, Gramma, just one more time," he said.

"Oh, Ben, you know I'd take you with me if I could," she said.

"Gramma, you can hug me good-bye if you want."

My mother hugged Ben and he hugged her back so hard it surprised even me. I saw my mother's eyes filling up with tears. She knew how much it hurt him. And she knew that this time, it was really good-bye.

"I'll always love you, Gramma," Ben said.

"I'll always love you too, Ben. Remember, you're the one who made me a gramma."

Ben turned to Ralph.

"I love you, too, Grampa," Ben said, hugging him. "Good-bye."

It was all Ralph could do to hold back his tears until they were outside.

Grant's parents came up the next day. Gramma Oyler sat outside with Ben in the yard for an hour or more, the two of them, just keeping company. And that evening, Grant and his dad read some scriptures to Ben.

Ben loved his grandparents. When they left, he watched from the living room until they were out of sight. Then he leaned over the heater vent by the living-room window, looking as forlorn as I'd ever seen him.

I went over and stood by him and resisted the urge to hug him.

He didn't say anything. He just leaned against me, held one arm up in the air, and let his hand come to rest around my neck. The Ben Hug. Ben's way in those last days of saying "I love you."

* * *

The next day the director of the home nursing service stopped by to see how things were going. We had nurses almost around the clock now. I think one of them had told her that Ben was nearing the end.

She talked about the duty schedule and asked if there was anything else we needed.

I hesitated for a moment and then I asked her, "Have you been around a lot of people who are dying?"

"Yes," she told me, she had.

"What should I expect? What's it like for them?"

She began by telling me that she had talked to a lot of patients who had been near death and had been brought back and they almost always told of the same experience.

"They say there's this really warm feeling that comes over them. And that they can feel their spirit leaving their body and being lifted up.

"They usually see a light. Some say it's a light at the end of a dark tunnel . . . others say it's like a bright light in the corner of a room . . . but always, always it's a light that is beckoning them . . .

"They feel torn. They want to follow the light but they don't want to leave the people they love behind.

"The best thing you can do for Ben is let him know that it's okay to go . . . okay to leave you. And that you love him."

10

"Go Toward the Light"

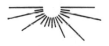

THE CLOCKS KEPT TICKING. The newspaper kept arriving at our front door every evening. And the weathermen kept predicting what the skies would look like the next day.

I wanted to stop time. I wanted to stop the very sun in the sky. But I couldn't. Three more days and it would be Friday, the Fourth of July.

For a couple of weeks now, ever since we had decided not to go back to the hospital, Grant and I had set aside two or three hours every afternoon just for Ben. Beau would play for a few hours with friends. Danny would be down for a nap. Aber was at my Mom's.

And, for a while, it was as if we had come full circle, back to the time when there was just Grant and me and Ben. Only now we weren't beginning our time together but ending it.

We would sit by the bed in Ben's room—that wonderful little-boy room full of sports posters and airplane models—and play a game or read stories, or sometimes just talk. It didn't matter, really. What mattered was that we were together.

"Mom, what do you think Jessica does in heaven all day?"

"I don't know, Ben, but I'm sure she's happy . . . you've been thinking a lot about Jessica lately, haven't you?"

"Um-hmm."

"You know, when you get to heaven, Jessica won't be

sick," Grant said. "She'll be just like all the other people. Everybody who was sick here will be well there. There is no disease, no illness, no affliction in heaven."

"Does that mean that when Uncle Scott dies he'll be able to see?"

"Yes, Ben, he will. Uncle Scott will finally get to see what you look like," I said.

"You won't be alone there, Ben. There'll be all sorts of people there to meet you. Remember Great-Grampa Boyle?"

"Sure, Dad. He always made me laugh . . . Dad, is it all right to laugh in heaven?"

Grant and I laughed.

"I don't see why not, Ben. I think Heavenly Father probably has a good sense of humor. He just might like the sound of people laughing," Grant said.

"You know, Ben, we don't know quite what the rules are up there," I said.

"You'll be the very first one from our family to go . . . but can you promise me something? Promise me that if there's any way you can, you'll come back to see us and tell us what it's like."

Ben gave me this quick little look that said he thought I knew better than that. And maybe I did . . . maybe.

"Okay, Mom. I promise."

❉   ❉   ❉

Ben was in a lot of pain that night. The medicine we were giving him never seemed to be enough. When Grant and I finally went to bed, I could hear the nurse opening the closet door, pulling the light chain, and closing the door over and over again as she repeatedly took out more medicine. Those sounds—the door, the light, and then the door again—engraved themselves in my memory.

Ben slept so little that night that he slept all the next morning. I could see from his face the toll that night had taken.

I called Judie and told her we needed to increase Ben's pain medicine. But she warned me that giving him much more could kill him or make him stop breathing. Finally, she consulted with Dr. Glader and called back to say we could increase the medicine a tiny fraction each hour. Eventually, she said, we would catch up with Ben's pain.

The house was very quiet as Ben continued to sleep. *This is what it will be like when Ben is gone,* I thought, *when his warm little spirit is absent.*

"What do you think about calling Ralph and asking if he would make Ben's casket?" Grant asked.

I thought about it for a minute. Ever since Ben was a baby, Ralph had spent time with him in his wood shop, sanding carousel horses, making birdhouses together.

"That would mean a lot to Ben. A whole lot," I said. "Let's call him."

Grant got my mother on the phone and asked her if she thought Ralph would be willing to do it.

"Hold on, I'll ask him," she said.

Grant could hear my mother and Ralph talking in the background. "You know what the kids are asking us to do, Ralph? They're asking us to put our arms around Ben in death the way we have in life."

Ralph came to the phone. He was emotional. This was a hard task for a grandfather, making a casket for his own grandson. He swallowed hard and answered, "I'll give it my best. What kind of wood do you want?"

"Pine," Grant said. "Something simple."

Ralph bought the wood and started to work that same day.

When Ben woke up that afternoon, we went in and sat with him. He was feeling a little better after his rest, but I could almost see the life force beginning to leave him.

"Dad?" he asked. "Can you give that to Grampa Oyler?"

I followed his gaze to the Pinewood Derby car on the desk.

"Sure, Ben," Grant said.

I could see Ben wanted to speak, but it was hard for him.

"Ben, have you ever heard of something called a will?" I asked.

He shook his head no.

"Well, sometimes when people die and they have a lot of people they love, they want to give them the things they have that are special. So they write it down. And they sign it. And that paper is called a will. Is that something you'd like to do?"

He nodded.

"How about if I point to things in your room that are

special, and you tell me who you want to give them to?" Grant said.

So Grant went around the room as I wrote.

There was something for everybody. The toy jeep you could actually ride in from the Make-a-Wish Foundation shopping spree. "For Aber."

Ben's wallet with nearly one hundred dollars in it. "For Jaap for school."

Something for his grandparents, his cousins, his brothers.

Tears began falling on Ben's journal as I was writing. And Grant brushed his own tears away with his arm, hoping Ben wouldn't notice. We couldn't help it, just listening to Ben give away the things that had mattered so much to him.

"I . . . don't . . . want you guys to be sad . . . okay?"

His voice was deep and hoarse. Grant and I looked at each other. This wasn't the way we wanted Ben to see us. We had come this far. We couldn't fall to pieces now. Not now.

"Okay, Ben," I said. "It's just that we'll miss you a lot, that's all."

"I'll miss you too," he said.

I leaned over and kissed him.

"Mom, you didn't ever sell my bike, did you?"

He was right. I hadn't. I had been hoping, just hoping that maybe someday . . .

"Write down my bike, Mom. For Beau."

When we finished, Ben signed his will, dated July 2, 1986. His signature was as simple as a child's and as frail as an old man's.

❧   ❧   ❧

That evening, Ben smelled popcorn popping on the stove, and asked to come out. So the nurse rolled his pumps to the living room and he sat there a while, just munching popcorn with Beau and watching TV, as if it were the most natural thing in the world.

But that night, the closet door opened and closed all night long.

"His pain was a ten most of the night," the nurse told me in the morning.

I sat with Ben that morning as we increased the pain medicine still more, a little each hour. His hourly dose seemed to take away the pain for only half an hour. And then I'd massage his arms and legs or try to talk to him to distract him from the pain until it was time for another dose.

Keeping my promise to Ben about not letting him die in pain was harder than I had ever imagined.

It wasn't until after dark on Thursday that the medicine finally caught up with Ben's pain. We were alone in his room, Ben and I. And it was quiet except for the gentle whooshing sound of his pumps.

"The veil is getting very thin for you now, isn't it, Ben?"

He nodded.

"Will it . . . hurt, Mom?"

I stroked his hair back from his forehead and kissed him.

"No, Ben. It won't hurt. Not anymore. I promise . . .

There's nothing for you to be afraid of, not now. It'll just feel like you're coming home from a long vacation. Remember? Only when you get home, it won't be to this house. But it will feel warm and comfortable, just like home.

"And . . . and, before you know it, Benny, we'll all be there with you. Dad and Beau and Aber and Danny and me. It'll feel like just the twinkling of an eye until we're all together again forever, Ben. That's how quick it will be. Just like a twinkling of an eye."

"I . . . love . . . you . . . , Mom," he said.

He closed his eyes and I just sat there, looking at his face and stroking his hair.

And I love you, Ben. I don't know what I'm going to do without you. I know that earth isn't a place to stay forever, just to be a while and then move on. But why, why are you leaving me so soon? Do you know? Have you already learned those lessons from life that take the rest of us decades to learn? Or does . . . does God have some special need for you in heaven, some divine mission for you to carry out there that we can't know?

I took Ben's hand in mine and held it. I put it up to my lips and gently kissed it. Then I noticed his fingers had a bluish cast.

I had heard that when people die, they die from the hands and feet up.

"It's close, isn't it?" I whispered to the nurse when she came in a few minutes later.

"Yes," she said. "Tonight, maybe, or tomorrow. It's hard to tell."

I told Grant. He came in and sat on Ben's bed, and Ben stirred, then opened his eyes.

"Ben . . . ," Grant began. "I just wanted to tell you that . . . that I feel honored to have you as my son."

Tears streamed down his face.

"I've tried to be a good father to you, to teach you right from wrong. But you're the one who's taught me. I wanted you to know that. You taught me so much. How to appreciate life while we're here. How to have faith, really have faith, even when you pray as hard as you can for a miracle and it doesn't happen, at least not the way you thought it would."

"Dad . . . Daddy, you don't have to . . . I know . . ."

But Grant went on. He couldn't stop his tears now, not even for Ben.

"You know, Ben, I always wanted to be a dad. All my life. Ever since I was a little boy like you. Then I married Mom and we had you, Ben. And we were so happy. You were so cute and we couldn't believe how blessed we were to have you. And I kept dreaming about all the things we'd do together . . . well, it looks like we're not going to get to do some of those things together now, Ben.

"And I'll miss that, son. Not a day will go by that I won't miss you. And Mom'll miss the flowers you give her and the letters you write. And Beau and Aber and Danny will miss you too. We'll all miss you, Ben.

"But, no matter how much we'll miss you, Ben, it's all right if you leave us. I mean that. I really do. But I couldn't let you just, just go. Without telling you . . . how much I love you and how much I'll miss you. But that part's built in, the missing each other. People who love each other miss each other when they're not together. They just do.

"But I don't want you to be afraid or to worry about us. We'll be all right. And you'll be fine, Ben. All this pain, it'll be gone. All gone. And we understand that you have to go. It's okay with us, Ben. Whenever you want to let go, we're ready . . ."

Grant leaned down on Ben's chest and Ben put his arms around him and held him. And he was crying.

"I love you, Dad," he said. "I love you . . . I love you."

Grant kissed Ben and left the room.

He could not bear to sit by our son's deathbed. And I could not bear to leave.

We were alone now, Ben and I. I knew we would be the last to say good-bye. And now our time had come. But we just looked into each other's eyes. Neither of us said a word. Then Ben squeezed my hand. His eyelids closed. And he fell asleep, deeply now. The medicine was taking hold. And I knew I had kept my promise.

*   *   *

How long has it been? More than a year now since that day we brought you home and you sat in my lap and we drew up that list of things you could look forward to. The Oyler reunion. Your baptism. The new house. School. I know you wanted to go to school, Ben. But wasn't what you really wanted from school a friend? And you got a friend, didn't you, Ben? Jaap was your friend, wasn't he?

Jessica . . . She was on your list too. And you'll get to see her soon now, Ben. When the veil lifts, I'm sure she'll be standing right there on the other side. She'll help you, Ben, if you need it. The way you helped her here.

So, didn't you get them all, Ben? All the things on the list you really wanted?

Yes, even a baby brother. Danny's a lot like you when you were a baby. He was God's gift to me, to all of us. I know that.

Your Dad and I got what we needed, too. Something we needed more than anything. Time. Time to learn from you how to be brave, how to make the best times of our lives out of our darkest days.

Time to be with you and love you and watch you grow strong inside, in your soul.

If I hadn't had that time to see the spiritual side of you growing, Ben, I don't know if I would have had the strength to pray to release your soul from this body. I don't know if I could have done it. Not a year ago . . . not even a month ago . . .

I couldn't have sat here, calmly watching you, taking in every breath, every flutter of your eyes. Are you dreaming, Ben? What do you see in your dreams now? Are you looking back, or are you looking ahead?

Oh, Ben, how I'll miss you.

But I'm not afraid . . . am I?

Just because I can't stop my tears doesn't mean I can't bear this. I have to cry, Ben. I'm your mother and nothing could ever hurt me again as much as losing you. You're a part of me. And when you leave, a part of me will go too. And after that, a part of me will always be missing, no matter if I live to be a hundred.

I can feel the hurt already, rising up from deep inside me and knotting in my throat. When you're gone and I feel lost, I'll remember how brave you were and take heart from you, Ben.

This is the one trial of faith I knew I could never bear. And yet I am bearing it. And even now, I can feel the warmth of the blessings that come after.

So your dad was right, Ben. Miracles do happen, they do.

❋   ❋   ❋

Ben woke with a start just before midnight.

"Where's Beau?" he asked.

"He's asleep in the other room. Do you want me to get him?" He didn't answer.

"Where's Aber?"

"At Gramma's."

"Where's Danny?"

"Asleep in his crib."

Then his eyes closed again and he went back to sleep.

The nurse came in and told me I'd better get some sleep myself. "You'll need your strength later," she said. Finally, I took her advice and went to bed. I asked her to call us if there was even the slightest change.

❋   ❋   ❋

Two of Ralph's woodworking students had volunteered to help him make the casket. The three of them worked virtually around the clock. They didn't know how much time was left.

It was two o'clock Friday morning when they finally finished. Exhausted, Ralph had climbed into bed next to my mom and had just fallen asleep when Aber came into their room and stood by their bed in the dark.

"Gramma, Gramma!" he said. "There's a little ghost flying around my room."

"Oh, Aber, honey, it's just a bad dream."

Aber shook his head back and forth.

"No, Gramma. It's a REAL ghost."

"Okay—would you feel better if I came in for a little while and lay down with you?"

Aber nodded and the two of them went back into Aber's room. After Aber was settled in my mother said to him, "See, Aber? There was no ghost, was there?"

"Yes, there was, Gramma. It was Ben. He came in here and told me that he won't have to hurt anymore 'cause he's got only one more day here.

"He told me he loved me and he'd miss me a lot."

*   *   *

It was almost 5:00 A.M. when Ben sat bolt upright in bed.

The nurse summoned us.

When we got to his room, Ben was lying back down again. His eyes were closed. I sat down on his right side, and

Grant sat beside me. I put my arms around him and whispered in his ear.

"Ben!" I whispered. "Mom and Dad are here and we love you, Ben. We love you so much."

His body was very tense in my arms, moving in odd little ways as if unsure what it was supposed to do.

"We'll miss you, Ben . . . We'll all miss you . . ."

I could feel his body relax very slightly, in my arms.

"Ben, do you see a light? A warm and comforting light? Follow it. It's there for you, Benny, to show you the way . . ."

I felt his body go limp in my arms and I felt the immense power of the pain he was releasing. His hand opened with his palm up on the bed. Instinctively I reached for it, the way I had when he was little, as if to stop him from falling.

Then, as quickly as my fear had come, it passed.

I sat back, and leaned against Grant.

The room was full of Ben. He was all around us, everywhere. Warm and loving. He was lingering there for a moment to say good-bye. To tell us not to worry, that there wasn't anything to be afraid of, and never was.

Go toward the light, Ben.

Go toward the light.

Epilogue

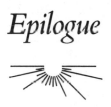

I SAID AT THE BEGINNING that helping Ben die was the hardest thing I would ever do. I know now that I was wrong. Harder by far was learning to live without him.

Ben died on July 4, 1986.

The awful emptiness set in the next day, the first day I had spent in nine years without Ben in it. I lay on his bed to remember the smell of Ben. I closed my eyes a dozen times to try to commit to memory the Ben expressions I loved.

We didn't want the formal ritual of a funeral for Ben. Instead, we wanted something to reflect our family, something to symbolize life. So rather than a hearse and a big, black limousine, we decided to put Ben's casket in the back of our white Toyota van. "Ben O" was carved in the top of the casket. And inside Grampa Ralph had put the little wooden whale Ben loved. Gramma Oyler had made the white satin lining.

Ben's cousins Brett, Joey, Sam, and Mike and my brothers, Steve and Randy, and Grant's brothers, Richard and Brian, were pallbearers. They carried the small casket inside the chapel for service.

The summer sun threw bright streams of light through the windows. The chapel was filled with flowers and people who loved Ben coming together to say good-bye.

Grampa Oyler said the eulogy, which had more to do with Pinewood Derbys and Ben's faith and his love of a little girl named Jessica than it did about death. And Grant spoke for a few minutes about his son. His voice was strong and proud. But tears were streaming down his face as he spoke.

At the end, we sang Ben's favorite song, "Families Are Forever." Everyone had to turn to their program after the first verse; Ben was the only one who knew all the words.

We buried our son on a sunny hill under a large oak tree. My dad, Bill Eckholdt, said the graveside dedication. When they lowered Ben's body into the ground, Beau and Aber leaned over and looked down into the grave after their brother.

I can still remember their faces, so serious and sad. Beau was the last one to look away.

❁   ❁   ❁

I told myself that pretty soon I'd have to do something with Ben's things, do something with the medicine and the clothes.

But it was painful just to open the closet door and switch on the light.

For a long time, Grant and I avoided doing "Ben things." Even now, Grant rarely plays golf. We went on short vacations and took photographs. But I had nine rolls of film in my purse before I could bring myself to have it developed. I couldn't bear the thought of getting back pictures without Ben in them.

For months, I couldn't seem to remember how to do the simplest things. When I went to set the table for dinner at night, I'd find I had taken out five settings of silverware and six plates. Strangers would ask how many children I had, and I'd start to say "four" and then stop.

I'd like to say that I found solace enough in my husband and other boys. But that wasn't really true, at least in the beginning. At first, there was a big gaping hole inside me that nobody could fill. But what I realized soon after Ben's death was that I had to get to know my own children and my husband all over again. We had learned to function in crisis, learned to love each other through tears. But now we had to learn how to function all over again in normal times, when alarm clocks went off in the morning and there was homework to do at night.

We are a new family now. We have a different eldest child. And we have a new baby brother who knows about Ben but who will never remember how much Ben loved him. When he heard us talking about Ben a few months ago, he held up his little baby hands and said, "All gone."

Starting over has been especially difficult for Beau. He didn't sleep well for months after Ben died, and often woke up with nightmares. He still does not consider himself the big brother. Whereas Ben was wry and thoughtful, Beau is open and direct, even blunt. As painful as it has been for him, I think he will grow up to be a more compassionate man for what he has been through.

To my joy, I discovered one day that Beau has an inclination toward art. And just as Ben was the leader of the pack at the Oyler reunions, Beau is now the leader of the pack at the Eckholdt reunions. Yes, we have reunions now. Ben's death has brought our family closer. My dad sometimes calls just to say hi and we get together often.

Grant responded to Ben's death by working. His business is doing well now. I'm proud of him. Particularly proud because when Bishop Rasband retired from his position, Grant was chosen to succeed him. People come to Grant for consolation and advice now the way we went to Dr. Rasband. They say he understands their problems—in his heart.

My mother, whom I turned to so often for help during our ordeal, lost her own son just over a year after Ben died. My brother Scott died of complications of his hemophilia, and we buried him next to Ben. As Ben said, he won't have to be blind anymore. I trust he and Ben are together.

As for me . . . I have had to learn how to be myself all over again. I had forgotten what I used to be like before Ben's illness. I couldn't remember what I used to do, or what words I used to say, or what people had expected of me, before Ben became ill. My old definition of myself as mother wasn't enough: my confidence in that role had been too shaken.

At first, there were things to do that revolved around Ben. There was the brass leaf to hang on the tree in the lobby of the Ronald McDonald House in memory of Ben. There was the tombstone—with the words "Go Toward the Light" at the top and "Families Are Forever" at the bottom—to put on Ben's grave.

Epilogue

Dr. Infelice, the superintendent of schools who had declined to enroll Ben in school, nominated me to the California State Board of Education's Advisory Committee on AIDS. He told *Newsweek* a year after Ben's death that if he had it to do over again, his decision would be different.

When those things, those "Ben things," were taken care of, I couldn't put it off anymore: I had to start a new life for myself and my family.

I started by making a list that began with "figure out what makes you happy." When I did, I came full circle, back to the things that had made me happy before. It happened one day when we were driving back in the van from a skiing trip. I looked around me and everyone was smiling and the sky was blue and the sun was bright and I couldn't see anything wrong.

That simple realization was an incredible comfort: nothing was wrong. I had tomorrow to spend with three bright little boys with freckles on their noses and a husband who loved me. Then, right before my eyes, that little black cloud, the one that had been parked over our house ever since Ben got sick, just disappeared.

I still think of Ben, of course I do. Though Ben isn't here, I am still his mother.

There's a word for a woman whose husband has died: *widow.* Why, I wonder, isn't there a term for a woman whose child has died? I suppose because you never stop being a mother . . . even when your child is gone. You carried that child inside you, and you participated in the miracle of life when that child was born. And you know that all that energy and love cannot just vanish without a trace.

So I know, because I am a mother, that life doesn't simply end. Life can change. It can be altered. It can take on a new shape and form. But it never simply ends.

I know Ben is still alive—in that place the light came from. I wonder what his days are like, if he has days. I hope the things we taught him have been useful.

I saw Ben once, in a dream. He was taller than he used to be, grown up, as if he had never been sick. He stood out in the middle of a crowd and I went to him. But, as I opened my arms for his embrace, he stepped back. "Don't you know, Mom?" he whispered. "You can't touch me here."

I don't know how I would ever have come to terms with Ben's death if I didn't believe in God. My faith, and Grant's, is stronger now. What we believed before in our heads, we live now, in our hearts.

One day I will see Ben again. I know I will. Just as I know our whole family will be together again. But, as I'm sure Ben could tell you, that doesn't mean I wouldn't give the world for a hug.